WHEN TO REFUSE TREATMENT

Joseph F. Bentivegna M.D.

MICHELLE PUBLISHING COMPANY

ROCKY HILL, CT 06067

Bentivegna, Joseph Francis, 1956-

When to Refuse Treatment
Includes Index

Copyright © 1992 by Joseph F. Bentivegna M.D.

ISBN 0-962-60011-3

DEDICATION

To my family and my patients.

ACKNOWLEDGMENTS

Many people aided in the formation of this book. I would like to thank Dr. Dennis Gabos, Dr. David Hoffman, Dr. Marie Monticciolo and Dr. Richard Monticciolo for their insightful suggestions. My patients, Mrs. Rhoda Abel and Mr. Stanton Abel gave me valuable pointers from the laypersons' point of view. The comments of Attorney Wanda Justesen greatly enhanced the accuracy of the first several chapters. The fastidious proofreading of Mrs. Vivian Amster improved the readability of the manuscript. The photography of Mr. Gene Little and the illustrations of Mr. Nicholas Bentivegna were greatly appreciated. I also would like to thank Mr. Martins O. Maidelis for his help in preparing the actuarial tables.

TABLE OF CONTENTS

PREFACE

The purpose of this book is quite simple. It is to show patients how to recognize when their condition is terminal, when they have lost their will to live and when they should consider refusing treatment. It is not to advocate euthanasia or suicide in the terminally ill, but merely a practical guide to steer patients and their families through the labyrinth of our legal and health care system while trying to pass away in peace.

Traditionally, physicians are trained to preserve life and relieve suffering. Unfortunately, the technological advances of the past decades often bring these goals into conflict. While the dying once spent their final days peacefully at home surrounded by family and friends, many now find themselves entwined in a mass of electrodes and wires while effete doctors solemnly peruse bloated charts replete with laboratory data confirming the obvious. Society is attempting to remedy the situation with a sundry of legal maneuvers such as living wills, medical directives and health care proxies. Yet patients already have the most important right: the right to refuse treatment. A recent law, The Patient Self-Determination Act, is the medical equivalent of the Miranda Law. Patients must be informed of their right to refuse treatment when they enter a hospital or nursing home. As this book will explain, asserting this right requires mostly common sense.

It is hoped this book will help to bring back a more genteel way of dying. Improved technology will soon usher in a home-health care revolution. Fax machines, miniature ultrasounds, video cameras and compact blood analyzers will allow doctors to provide home care with the same efficiency presently provided in hospitals. Intravenous antibiotics, chemotherapy and pain medication may also be given at home. The problem is that the health care establishment has not yet become enamored with home-health care and reimbursement for this service is still limited. Nonetheless, many patients are asserting themselves and refusing hospitalization when they believe their condition is terminal. This is the way it used to be until doctors, hospitals, judges and lawyers intervened.

Since dying is generally the province of the elderly, their problems are discussed in an appropriately proportionate manner. Nonetheless, anyone can benefit from reading this book, especially those entrusted with caring for the elderly and younger persons afflicted with terminal cancer and AIDS.

INTRODUCTION

During medical school, one of my professors climbed on his soap box and righteously intoned that as physicians, we should never take hope away from a patient. This is the way doctors are trained. Death is our failure. Yet every human being born dies. While theologians may wish to cite several exceptions, few would refute this. Unfortunately, our medical technology has evolved more rapidly than has our wisdom. Just as nuclear weapons have given humanity destructive power undreamed of 100 years ago, society is now forced to grapple with ethical issues that were previously inconceivable. Patients used to be afraid of dying; now they are afraid of not dying. They are afraid they will be connected to machines that prolong their lives indefinitely. They are afraid they will be squirreled away in nursing homes – sedated and restrained – while their life savings are depleted, their dignity stripped, and their children are forced to tend to their needs.

Recent court cases have brought the issue of life-prolonging treatment to the front pages. In the case of Karen Anne Quinlan, a state court ruled that a respirator (a machine that breathes for the patient) may be removed from a comatose patient. The Supreme Court ruled in the Cruzan case that a feeding tube could be removed from a comatose patient if evidence existed that the patient did not desire her life to be prolonged artificially. Yet these instances are rare. The more common scenario is that of an elderly family member slowly losing the ability to handle her affairs and having difficulty performing the activities of daily living such as driving a car, taking a bath, going to the bathroom, shopping and feeding herself.

My grandmother's death is one reason for my decision to write this book. The quintessential Italian grandmother, she was an 80-year-old picture of health with the exception of being overweight from the ingestion of her outstanding cooking. Her doctor had prescribed a diuretic for high blood pressure, but she refused to take it because it made her urinate often. While walking in her house, she suddenly had

3

a throbbing headache and fainted. A quick call brought the ambulance and an adept emergency room doctor intubated her (placed a breathing tube in her throat) and put her on a respirator. She lost consciousness and a CAT scan (a sophisticated X-ray) of her head revealed that she had a ruptured aneurysm.

With aggressive treatment, it was theoretically possible that the blood in my grandmother's brain would resorb and she would return to rolling meatballs and advising her grandson the doctor to look both ways before crossing the street. What would more likely happen is that she would have remained in a coma indefinitely — paralyzed and wearing diapers. As Medicare (the program that provides partial health insurance to the disabled and those over 65) does not fund long-term care, her life savings would have been rapidly depleted. As one of her prayers had been for a quick death, she undoubtedly would have found this outcome repulsive.

My family, especially my aunt and uncle who still lived with her, were devastated. Nobody wanted to see my grandmother die and I explained as diplomatically as I could that she had already died. Removing the respirator that was keeping her body alive would have unleashed a family battle that would pale Gettysburg. Fortunately there was another option — refusing further treatment. This option was eloquently enunciated by Justice Benjamin Cardozo in 1914. "Every human being of adult years and sound mind has a right to determine what shall be done with his own body." If she could not decide, her family could. Her doctor gave us the option of placing a feeding tube in her stomach. I doubt if the doctor would have done this to his grandmother, but he was obligated to mention it. After considerable persuasion on my part, I convinced my family this was not a wise move. Several days later, my grandmother's heart stopped beating.

As a physician, I understood the ramifications of placing a feeding tube and permitting resuscitation. Although my other family members were well-educated, having never experienced this dilemma before, they would have made a disastrous decision. But what happens to families who do not understand the consequences of these aggressive interventions?

Patients trying to die in peace routinely bombarded the emergency room of the hospital where I interned. Typically, the patient was a

4

comatose nursing home denizen in her late eighties who was being kept alive by a feeding tube. Attired in a hospital gown and diapers, she would have a catheter (a tube for incontinent patients) inserted into her genital area as she had long lost the ability to control her excretory functions. While in the hospital, the family would place an old picture of her beside her bed, perhaps to remind her caretakers that this 80-pound contracted skeleton was once a functioning member of society who raised a family, went to church on Sunday and voiced her opinions at the local PTA meetings. I wondered what the patient would have said if I could turn back time and ask her if she wanted to be prolonged in this condition. Several months into my internship, I vowed that no patients assigned to me that were trying to die in peace would have a feeding tube placed.

My approach was simple. I merely explained to the family that no feeding tube could be placed without their permission. This was news to them. They just assumed that if some white coat waltzed into their loved one's room and said it was necessary, they had to agree and meekly sign the requisite form. Many were concerned that their loved one would die without this tube. I explained that although I did not have a crystal ball, it was unlikely that any treatment would return their loved one to health. In all likelihood, she would languish in the nursing home contracting recurrent infections while the tube kept her alive. Eventually, a heart attack or stroke would take her, but this could take years. Given this information, no family ever consented to having a feeding tube placed.

This sad state of affairs has happened rapidly, in only twenty to thirty years. While many reasons may be cited, there are two major ones. The first is that medical technology has increased rapidly, permitting doctors to keep patients alive when they are trying to die. The second is that our increasingly litigious society has shell-shocked doctors into abandoning common sense and aggressively treating the dying to avoid lawsuits.

The major life-prolonging treatments are feeding tubes, cardiopulmonary resuscitation (CPR), antibiotics, and respirators. The injudicious use of these treatments often results in a macabre contracted skeleton that no one can rationally justify. Yet, predicting these horrendous outcomes is impossible with 100% accuracy. There will always be episodes of a healthy individual who has a heart attack and is resuscitated only to suffer permanent brain damage. Nonetheless, those with terminal diseases who have lost their will to live can prevent having their lives vainly prolonged if they assert themselves. The key is to become an educated consumer.

While the slow engines of government are finally digesting the rapid technological advances that have created these dilemmas, legislative initiatives can never replace personal control. Living wills may afford you some protection, but they can be contested or ignored. Many patients who sign living wills do not realize that in most states, a doctor can override them with impunity. Even as legislation and court decisions allow the removal of feeding tubes and respirators, the bureaucracy of having this done can be time-consuming, expensive and emotionally draining. The strongest protection exists right now — the right to refuse treatment. Thus, in spite of all the changes in the legal and ethical milieu, the best way to avoid having your life prolonged is to understand your condition and assert yourself. If you are unable to do so, make sure a family member or friend knows your wishes and has a strong enough personality to do what has to be done.

NOTES AND ASIDES

This book is not meant to replace the advice of a physician. Each patient is unique, each disease is different and there are exceptions to every rule. Always make medical decisions on when to refuse treatment in concert with a physician, not unilaterally.

*   *   *

There are literally thousands of lethal diseases. This book centers on the most common ones. The biggest killers in the United States are listed below.

DISEASE	PERCENTAGE OF DEATHS
Heart disease	38%
Strokes/Alzheimers	8%
Lung Cancer	8%
Other Cancers	15%
Emphysema	4%
Pneumonia	2%
Accidents	5%
AIDS	1%
Others	19%

Statistics are given throughout the book regarding the mortality rate of various diseases. While this may be obvious to most readers, permit me to define some concepts. Five-year survival means the percentage of people alive after five years. For example, the 5-year survival in patients with lung cancer is 12%. This means that in 100 patients with newly-diagnosed lung cancer, 12 will be alive in five years. Average life span is simply the average of all time periods patients live after a given diagnosis. For example, a patient with newly-diagnosed lung cancer has an average life span of nine months.

*   *   *

In fin de siècle America, it has become verboten to use only masculine pronouns generically. The English language has not evolved to the level of Creole, in which their are no masculine and feminine pronouns. Constantly writing "he or she" and "himself or herself" is cumbersome. Thus I randomly use either the masculine or feminine pronouns throughout this book. I hope readers do not find it confusing.

CHAPTER 1

DYING AND
PROLONGING LIFE

As an ophthalmologist, I commonly diagnose cataracts that are too small to warrant surgery. I inform the patient that in five years, surgery may be necessary when the vision diminishes to the point where it impedes her lifestyle. Invariably, she replies "Oh I'll be dead by then."

In fact the overwhelming likelihood is that she will not be dead. The favorable economic conditions and the improved medical care of the twentieth century have resulted in an unprecedented increase in life span. The average life span in ancient Rome was 22 years and in India in 1900, those who lived to be 20 were ahead of the game. Alexander the Great had conquered the entire known world by age 32. In 1915 the average life span was 54 years in the United States. Now it is 74 and still climbing (see Figure 1-1). Every two years, the average life span increases by four months. Years ago, 60-year wedding anniversaries were a rarity but now they are routine and there is no paucity of centenarians for Willard Scott to salute.

What has not changed, though, is the maximum life span. Even in ancient Rome, rare individuals lived into their hundreds. Human

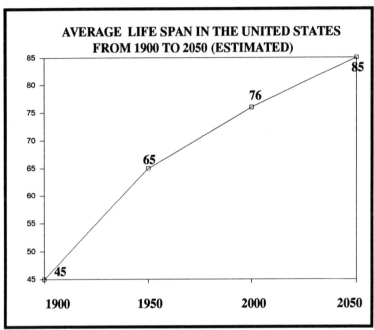

Figure 1-1

longevity is limited by the number of times a human cell can accurately reproduce — the so-called Hayflick Principle. Perhaps the best way to explain this is by an everyday example. If you duplicate the key to your car, use the new key to make another copy and continue this process several times, eventually a key is created that will not start the car. With a sophisticated key-copier, this may occur after 50 duplications, but with an older model, it may happen after only 30 duplications. The same phenomenon occurs with cell division in the human body and the maximum number of replications varies from individual to individual. This limits the maximum life span in most humans to between 80 and 90 years although some individuals with the right DNA live to be over 100.

Please take a look at Figure 1-2. This chart shows the average life span at a given age according to sex. For example, the average life span of a 10-year-old boy is 73 while that of a 40-year-old woman is 80. This

AVERAGE LIFE SPAN FOR A GIVEN AGE

Age	Male	Female	Age	Male	Female
0	72	78	85	90	91
10	73	79	86	91	92
20	73	80	87	92	93
30	74	80	88	93	94
35	74	80	89	94	95
40	75	80	90	95	96
45	75	81	91	96	96
50	76	81	92	97	97
55	77	82	93	97	98
60	78	83	94	98	98
65	80	84	95	99	99
70	82	85	96	100	100
75	84	87	97	100	101
76	85	87	98	101	101
77	85	87	99	102	102
78	86	88	100	103	103
79	86	88	101	103	104
80	87	89	102	104	104
81	87	89	103	105	105
82	88	90	104	106	106
83	89	90	105	107	107
84	90	91			

How to read this chart - Simply look up a given age and read the average life span according to sex. For example, an 80-year-old woman on the average lives to be 89. An 86-year-old man on the average lives to be 91.

Figure 1-2

is not esoteric knowledge and is used by insurance companies to calculate pension benefits, health insurance costs and life insurance premiums. Notice that women live longer than men although the difference in life span decreases with increasing age. Sixty-five percent of those over 85 are women.

The key point is that the older you get, the greater the chance that you will exceed the average life span. While this may seem absurdly obvious, few actually understand its ramifications. For example, a male born today has an average life span of 72; however, a man who is 50 years old today on the average will live to be 76. Frequently, a patient's daughter, who is 57 years old, will inform me she plans to "enjoy life" when her 80-year-old mother succumbs. But look at Figure 1-2 under female. Her mother on the average will live another nine years and as can be seen from the more detailed longevity chart in Appendix 1, has a 19% chance of living to be 95. The daughter will be a senior citizen by the time the mother passes away!

Old age has traditionally been defined as 65 but this is a remnant of earlier times. In 1935 when Social Security was enacted, 65 was the average life span. However, today 85% of people 65 years old have no physical problems. Again, look at the chart in Figure 1-2 and you will see that a 65-year-old woman on the average lives to be 84. In a sense, improved medical technology and healthier lifestyles have created a second middle age, from 50 to 75 years old. The number of golfers who can shoot below their age is increasing every day. A major result of this trend is the increased time people are willing to work. Corporate executives, college professors and judges are legally challenging the concept of mandatory retirement, seeing no reason why they should discontinue a career they love because of some arbitrary age.

Even royalty cannot escape this trend. Many heirs apparent will have to wait most of their lives until they ascend the throne. Take, for example, the case of when Prince Charles will become king. His mother Queen Elizabeth II is now 65 and he is 42 (in 1991). She has a 50% chance of living to be 84 but remember, the Queen Mother is now a healthy 90. While the Queen inherited the right to rule the British Empire, it is also possible she inherited longevity. There is a very good chance that she will live to be 91 and if she does not choose to abdicate, Prince Charles may not become king until his late sixties!

But the major demographic change in the United States is the huge increase in people over the age of 85, the fastest growing segment of the population. In 1960, there were 2,700,000 but by 1985 the number of people over 85 had more than doubled to 5,600,000 (Figure 1-3). Furthermore by 2030, over 12,000,000 Americans will be 85 or older.

There is a huge difference in the level of function of a 70-year-old when compared to the level of function of an 85-year-old. Yet society tends to list both of these groups into one monolith called the elderly. It is those 85 and older – the super-elderly – who often lose control of their lives due to mental incompetence or physical disability. Also, the

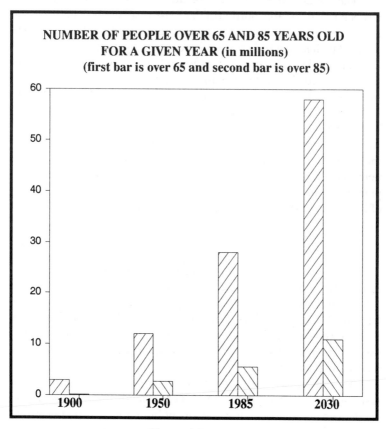

Figure 1-3

super-elderly, even when in ostensibly good health, often have difficulties with the activities of daily living. The burden of care for these people falls mostly on daughters and daughters-in-law. It has given rise to a "sandwich generation" of women who must care for their parents just after they have finished raising their children. It is equivalent to a full-time job, as the super-elderly need help bathing, eating, and going to the bathroom. Many are unable to drive and require transportation to the doctor's office, laboratories, X-ray facilities, supermarkets and social events. The lives of many of the super-elderly can easily be prolonged by medical technology.

The political and social reverberations of increased longevity are just beginning. A large portion of the massive amounts of government and corporate debt is due to the fact that no one anticipated that medical technology and improved economic assistance to the elderly would result in such rapid increases in life span. Many corporations who promised their retirees cost-of-living adjustments in their pensions and health care coverage now have hoards of red-faced actuaries who grossly underestimated these costs. While car companies like to blame the Japanese for their decreased sales, a large portion of the sticker price goes to funding health insurance policies and pensions of their retirees. Government service jobs and military careers, where people often retire in their forties and fifties, now must have pension plans that can ante up enough money to ensure a reasonable standard of living and health care coverage for 40 years!

*   *   *

The aging process is not sudden but gradual. While aging is thought by many to commence at 40, it actually starts earlier. There is a big difference in the body of a 20-year-old and a 35-year-old. In basketball, football and baseball, those who are 30 are considered to be cagy veterans and those who continue to play after age 35 are exceedingly rare and make a fortune hawking arthritis medicine and Geritol on television.

All functions—cardiovascular, visual, sexual, muscular and respiratory— gradually decrease with age (Figure 1-4). While physical deficits are annoying, it is the loss of brain function that destroys one's quality of life. Being relegated to a nursing home is more often

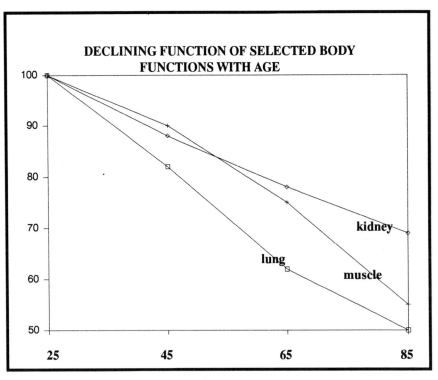

Figure 1-4

the result of mental rather than physical disabilities. Unlike physical function, though, a decrease in brain function is not inevitable with age. Some aspects do decline. For example, the ability to perform complex mathematical problems decreases. Many theoretical physicists and mathematicians do their best work in their twenties. Chess champions are usually over the hill by age 30. On the other hand, the ability to perform applied skills such as medicine and law does not decline. Many judges, doctors, lawyers and accountants reach their professional peak at age 50 and remain there.

*　　　*　　　*

Until recently, virtually everyone died rapidly and even today, most people die relatively quickly. Twenty-five percent of heart attack victims die within 48 hours in spite of well-equipped ambulances, readily-available modern emergency rooms, well-trained doctors and a high percentage of the lay population familiar with cardiopulmonary resuscitation (CPR). For most, death is not a horrible ordeal. A recent study by the National Institute of Aging revealed that over 50% of people die in their sleep. Eighty per cent were free of pain during the year before their death and 61% were pain free on their day of death.

Until the advent of modern medicine, those who did not have an instantaneous death still died relatively quickly. Patients debilitated by strokes, massive heart attacks and cancer contracted infections or developed kidney failure, conditions that proved fatal when nature took its course.

If you are a debilitated patient, you need to differentiate between the methods of prolonging life from the ways of comforting life (Figure 1-5). You have the choice of refusing any treatment unless the situation arises where you lose consciousness.

WAYS OF PROLONGING LIFE

1. Antibiotics. While more dramatic ways of prolonging life such as cardiopulmonary resuscitation, heart surgery and feeding tubes receive publicity, by far the most common way to keep a patient alive is by antibiotics. There is no close second. Invented only 50 years ago, antibiotics now cure previously common killers such as pneumonia and wound infections. During the Civil War and World War I, a soldier shot in the abdomen always died due to infection, even if no vital organs were injured. Two presidents, James Garfield and William McKinley would have survived assassination attempts if antibiotics had been available. As a matter of fact, the assassin of President Garfield claimed he only shot the president, his doctors killed him. He was right. President Garfield died from an infection that complicated the surgical attempt to remove the bullet. Had his doctors simply left the shrapnel in his body, he may have survived.

The first antibiotic was Penicillin but today there are literally hundreds. When used alone or in combination, they are capable of

16

WAYS OF PROLONGING LIFE	WAYS OF COMFORTING LIFE
1. Antibiotics 2. Surgery 3. Artificial Hydration 4. Artificial Nutrition 5. Cardiopulmonary Resuscitation (CPR) 6. Mechanical Ventilation 7. Chemotherapy and Radiation Therapy 8. Kidney Dialysis	1. Surgery 2. Pain Control 3. Chemotherapy and Radiation Therapy

Figure 1-5

eradicating all but the most fulminant infections. Thus many patients trying to die in peace are prolonged. During a rotation as a medical student, I was placed under the tutelage of a physician who cared for comatose patients. As they were sedentary and incontinent, infections were frequent. One patient had the type of infection that responded to the antibiotic Gentamycin, but my preceptor administered Penicillin instead. As a lowly medical student, I had no intention of questioning his judgement until he asked me why he chose Penicillin. I responded that perhaps laboratory studies of which I was unaware, indicated Penicillin was the best drug. He replied that he chose the wrong drug on purpose so the patient would succumb. He felt that if he did not treat the infection, his intentions would become obvious to the other health care professionals caring for the patient. To this day, I do not know why he confided in me. Perhaps he inaccurately assessed me as being shrewd enough to ascertain his motives anyway.

A large killer of the elderly is pneumonia and it was once termed "the old man's friend" as it made for a quick death in dying patients before the invention of antibiotics. Sir William Osler, a giant in medicine at the turn of the century, stated that pneumonia allowed the elderly to escape "those cold gradations of decay that make the last state of all so distressing." Patients who become incontinent to urine often have catheters placed in their genital areas to prevent them from soiling themselves. These catheters cause bladder and kidney infections that are lethal unless treated with antibiotics. Thus a patient who feels death is a blessing should consider refusing antibiotic treatment.

2. Chemotherapy/radiation therapy. These options are discussed in greater detail in Chapter 8. Basically, these modalities attack cancer cells by inhibiting their replication. There are two problems with this. First, they rarely eradicate all cancer cells and secondly, normal cells are also damaged, causing side effects. Thus, if these treatments are going to prolong life for several uncomfortable months, refusing them should be considered. Most oncologists (cancer specialists) are realistic about the benefits of chemotherapy and radiation therapy and do not give their patients false hopes. As a matter of fact, physicians themselves frequently refuse treatment when diagnosed with cancer.

3. Cardiopulmonary Resuscitation (CPR). This is an attempt to revive a heart that has either stopped beating or is beating too inefficiently to maintain a blood pressure compatible with life. This term is also applied to restarting respiratory function when, for example, a person is drowning.

There are vast differences in the levels of CPR depending on the expertise of the individuals performing it and the equipment available. For example, if you are eating in a restaurant and have a heart attack, an individual trained in CPR will perform chest compressions and breath into your mouth.

In a hospital setting or when being cared for by an ambulance crew, the first thing done is to see if you are breathing spontaneously. If not, you are then intubated, the process by which a tube is placed in your windpipe so that air can be pumped into your lungs with greater efficiency. An intravenous line is then placed and electrodes are put on your chest to monitor the electrical activity of your heart. Depending on the pattern seen, drugs, electrical stimulation of the heart (cardioversion) or both are given. If your caretakers are unable to establish a strong enough heart contraction to maintain a respectable blood pressure, they will perform chest compressions. When viewed by a lay person, CPR appears quite barbaric. CPR has been administered for over two decades and considerable data has been amassed regarding its efficacy. It is one of the most overrated procedures in medicine. CPR is defined as successful not only if the patient survives the episode, but also if the patient is discharged from the hospital alive. Using this definition, only 4 percent of patients over 70 survive CPR. Of this small percentage, many are permanently brain-damaged. Patients with pneumonia, AIDS, acute strokes and metastatic cancer almost never survive CPR. On the other hand, patients whose hearts stop because of an allergic reaction, drug overdose or trauma are saved by CPR. Patients can refuse CPR by asking their physician to classify them as DNR (do not resuscitate). Thus if you have a terminal or debilitating disease and do not wish to undergo CPR, inform your physician. Your intentions will be respected as long as you put it in writing.

In a non-health-care setting such as your home or a restaurant, the situation is more complicated. If you call an ambulance, highly-trained technicians will attempt to revive you. A scenario can develop in which you are having chest pain or difficulty breathing and then have an arrest after you have called them. These people may not accept a living will even if you put it in front of their faces. Some states permit patients to wear bracelets stating they do not desire CPR, but if you consider death to be a blessing, avoid calling an ambulance.

4. Mechanical ventilation. Once a patient is intubated, he is placed on a respirator. This machine has a sundry of settings that enable doctors to control the rate of breathing, the volume of air per breath, and the percent of oxygen in each breath. Because of media sensation, much of the lay public views being placed on a respirator as a permanent step. It isn't. As the patient's condition improves, an attempt is made to "wean" the patient by gradually reducing the breathing rate and then removing the breathing tube.

The respirator has saved countless lives, especially young children with asthma attacks and premature babies with underdeveloped lungs. It has also led to difficult medical situations where doctors and families have been reluctant to pull the plug. As will be discussed in Chapter 3, turning off a respirator is permitted in most states under certain circumstances. Mechanical ventilation was the focus of the Karen Ann Quinlan case. This unfortunate young lady became comatose after a drug and alcohol overdose and presumably was being kept alive by a respirator. The New Jersey Supreme Court permitted the family to have the respirator removed. Ms. Quinlan remained in a coma but breathed on her own for over a decade until she died.

5. Artificial nutrition. The loss of appetite has been known to be a sign of declining health since the time of Hippocrates. Doctors are so attuned to this symptom that they will suspect illness in a patient who loses weight, even if the patient claims to be dieting.

A patient unable to ingest food can be fed with liquid food in several ways:

> Intravenous nutrition (hyperalimentation)
> Nasogastric tube
> Gastrostomy tube - inserted into the stomach surgically
> Jejunostomy tube - inserted into the intestine surgically

The intravenous method — hyperalimentation — is expensive, costing up to $300 a day. It cannot be continued indefinitely either because the veins collapse or the kidneys and liver rebel and stop processing the liquid food. When food is given into the digestive tract, a tube (nasogastric tube) is inserted into the nose and passed down into the stomach. This tube is only temporary, because it irritates the nasal tissue, and must be replaced with a feeding tube inserted directly into the stomach or intestines through an abdominal incision.

In blockage of the digestive tract and when recovering from a debilitating operation, artificial nutrition can provide valuable time and calories to facilitate recovery. More often than not, though, patients are given artificial nutrition because they have no appetite, and in terminal cases, this often unnecessarily prolongs life. A patient in a coma can survive for decades with a feeding tube in the stomach and "competent" medical care.

6. Artificial hydration. This is often incorrectly classified with artificial nutrition. The human body can survive for weeks without food, but it will not last for three days without water. This is why political activists go on hunger strikes but not thirst strikes. They would be dead before their plight was publicized. Artificial hydration is usually given intravenously although it can be given through a nasogastric tube or a stomach tube.

7. Kidney dialysis. The twice-a-week sojourn to the dialysis center has become a ritual for tens of thousands of Americans. The kidneys are necessary both to excrete the poisonous by-products of our metabolism and to maintain the proper amount of fluid in our vascular system. When they stop functioning, death occurs within days unless the patient consents to dialysis.

Refusing dialysis is quite common. Of an estimated 80,000 patients on dialysis in a given year, 12,000 succumb by refusing continued dialysis.

8. Surgery. A dying patient may be inclined to refuse all surgery but this is not always a wise move. Surgery can often prevent painful situations and enhance one's quality of life. Recently, I was asked to see a patient dying of metastatic breast cancer who was having trouble reading. She was able to read with a bright lamp and a magnifying glass but had to read slowly. I told her that cataract surgery would probably improve her eyesight but that in her weakened state, she may heal slowly. She opted to make do, the correct decision because she passed away two months later. On the other hand, I operated on a man dying of lung cancer who had such large cataracts he could not enjoy television or read. He enjoyed 20/20 vision until he died a year later. In general, dying patients should consider surgery that will improve their quality of life or relieve pain.

*　　*　　*

There is no magic formula for knowing when to refuse treatment but common sense is just as important as medical knowledge. The factors that must be considered are: whether or not the patient is terminal, whether the patient is self-aware — and in debilitated patients — whether the patient has a will to live (Figure 1-6).

Throughout this chapter, the term terminal disease has been glibly bantered around without defining it. In a philosophical sense, we are

```
┌─────────────────────────────────────────────────────────────┐
│                                                               │
│   Major factors in determining whether to refuse treatment:   │
│                                                               │
│        1. Terminal versus non-terminal condition              │
│        2. Self-awareness                                      │
│        3. Will to live in debilitated patients                │
│                                                               │
│                                                               │
└─────────────────────────────────────────────────────────────┘
```

Figure 1-6

all terminal but for practical purposes, a terminal disease is one that cannot be cured with present medical technology such as AIDS or metastatic lung cancer. A non-terminal disease is a cold or a broken bone. In between is a huge gray area that includes diseases such as heart disease and emphysema. Depending on the circumstances, these entities may be terminal or non-terminal.

Self-awareness is the ability to think, appreciate one's surroundings, enjoy life and communicate with others. A patient can have gradations of self-awareness ranging from being comatose to being completely coherent. The loss of this precious commodity is the most feared complication of old age and many patients would prefer death as an alternative. On the other hand, those born mentally handicapped are generally content and should be given aggressive treatment unless they have a terminal condition.

Patients who are non-terminal and self-aware can be so physically debilitated that they lose their will to live (Figure 1-7). For example, a patient with a stroke or spinal cord injury may be paralyzed. Another patient may be so short of breath from emphysema that he is unable to walk to the bathroom. The dependency these entities engender often cause despair and loss of will to live.

There is a wide variation in the willingness of patients to tolerate physical disability. Men who did physical labor all their lives are much more psychologically devastated by limited mobility than those who performed intellectual endeavors. The late Senator Javits of New York who was noted for his intellectual prowess, was crippled by Lou Gehrig's disease. This not only bound him to a wheelchair but also required him to carry a portable ventilator. Yet he continued to write

```
┌─────────────────────────────────────────────────┐
│                                                 │
│         SIGNS OF LOSS OF WILL TO LIVE           │
│                                                 │
│      1. Patient states "I want to die."         │
│      2. Poor appetite and weight loss           │
│      3. Incontinence                            │
│      4. No purpose in life                      │
│                                                 │
└─────────────────────────────────────────────────┘
```

Figure 1-7

and lecture until the final weeks of his life. On the other hand, if he had suffered a stroke that resulted in poor memory, he probably would have lost his will to live in short order. Debilitated patients can decide for themselves if they want aggressive treatment. Doctors can give patients an idea as to their prognosis; however, only the patients can decide whether to keep fighting or to throw in the towel.

*   *   *

How does a doctor know when a patient has lost his will to live. Sometimes the signs are subtle but at other times, it is quite obvious. (Figure 1-7).

1. Patient states "I want to die." This is the most common and most often ignored sign. These poor patients are often subjected to tests and aggressive procedures against their will. Many are often diagnosed as having "depression." Every year or so, some study berates the medical profession for not treating the elderly more aggressively for depression. What must be realized is that many people are depressed for a good reason. For example, if a man losses his wife in an accident, one does not have to be a psychiatrist to understand why he is depressed. The cure for his depression is to wave a magic wand and and bring back his wife. Medications can only tide him over until he learns to deal with his grief. The same applies to an incontinent 85-year-old man sitting alone in a nursing home confined to a wheel chair. He has good reason to be depressed. The cure for his depression is to give him a new body, not some silly pill. If he states he wants to be left alone, his doctors and family should respect his decision. That's his right. Giving him antidepressants or having him declared incompetent is rarely if ever in his best interests.

2. Poor appetite and weight loss. The non-deliberate loss of weight is an accurate sign of impending death. Often misguided doctors and families force artificial nutrition on these patients. This may prolong an otherwise peaceful death.

3. Incontinence. There is Haitian proverb that states: "A man who soils himself will surely die." There are medical reasons why individuals may occasionally defecate and urinate on themselves—poor bladder tone or diarrhea. By and large though, a patient with no obvious reason who repeatedly loses continence is sending a message. He wants to be left alone to die in peace.

4. No purpose in life. People who have lost a sense of purpose in life often lose their will to live. It is well-documented that idle retirees have shorter life spans than those who continue to work. Companionship is also important. A single man with a dog lives longer than a single man without one. Divorced men living their final years alone die at a much earlier age. As a matter of fact, an unattached divorced man in his fifties has a worse prognosis than a cigarette smoker the same age. People in the midst of creative endeavors, waiting for their last child to marry, or aiding a dying spouse remain in remarkably good health. Corporation heads, Supreme Court justices, influential politicians, writers and artists amaze people half their age with their vitality. These individuals are high on life. Rarely does one hear of an elderly world leader dying suddenly. Ronald Reagan was the picture of health during the eight years of his presidency and departed the presidency at age 78. His doctors were flabbergasted by his recuperative powers when he sailed through surgery after the attempt on his life. George Bush is 66, technically a senior citizen ready to be on Medicare. Yet he is rarely portrayed as elderly and probably does not

24

consider himself to be so. These people rarely die until the Hayflick Principle becomes operative.

*　　*　　*

Given this information, it is possible to construct some general guidelines regarding whether or not to refuse treatment:

1. A patient with a terminal disease or a disease that is stealing his self-awareness should consider refusing treatment unless it makes him more comfortable or improves his quality of life.

2. Debilitated patients who do not have a terminal disease and are self-aware should accept treatment until they have lost their will to live.

Notice how will to live is not a factor in deciding treatment for terminal diseases and diseases that seize self-awareness. Every doctor treats noble patients who plan to "lick" their metastatic lung cancer or AIDS. With present technology, they are never successful. Everyone with these entities dies and aggressive treatment at best gives several months of life that may be degrading and painful. Non-terminal but debilitated patients should be given the option to refuse treatment.

SUMMARY

Life span is constantly increasing and many people are going to live well into their eighties and nineties. The aging process is not sudden but gradual, with many people losing their ability to function in their final years. There are several methods for prolonging life, the most common and effective being antibiotics.

Patients with terminal diseases and diseases that steal their self-awareness should consider refusing aggressive treatment. Those with slowly debilitating diseases should refuse treatment when they have lost their will to live. This is manifested by stating "I want to die," incontinence, poor appetite and weight loss and is more common among those who have lost their purpose in life.

Chapter 2

FINANCIAL ASPECTS OF TERMINAL CARE AND DYING

While many may find it distasteful to discuss money in a book about dying, it must be done. A big issue for the elderly is control and control means money. Money enables you to live independently, pay taxes on your house, hire drivers and house cleaners, and pay health care bills. While insurance policies may be necessary, insurance companies are always looking for an excuse not to pay, especially when their brilliant forays into junk bonds and real estate have rendered their stock as marketable as Saddam Hussein T-shirts. Thus in terminal care, cash is king.

The good news is that twentieth-century America is one of the few countries that has allowed its middle class to acquire significant assets. The bad news is, trying to retain these assets and pass them on to your heirs, while side-stepping the land mines of estate taxes and the cost of long-term health care requires expert advice and luck. Thirty percent of the money spent on health care in a person's life is spent in her final 40 days.

The purpose of this chapter is not to teach all the nuances of terminal-care financing, but merely to make you think about these issues so that you may consult an expert in the area. References are given so that you may further investigate areas that are pertinent to your life. A good starting point is to contact an attorney from:

The National Academy of Elder Law Attorneys
1730 East River Road, Suite 107
Tucson, AZ 85718.
602-881-4005

*   *   *

Anyone who wants to control his death must have control of his life. Thus, five things must be considered in anticipation of one's death:

1. Health insurance
2. Cost of long-term care, if needed
3. Taxes due on your estate upon your death
4. The disbursement of your estate upon your death
5. The handling of your financial affairs in the event you become incapacitated

HEALTH INSURANCE

Health insurance in the United States is truly a potpourri, but most elderly fall into one of three categories:

1. Medicare with private insurance
2. Medicare without private insurance
3. Medicare with Medicaid

By and large, you are protected from large hospital and doctor bills by Medicare. It is fashionable to complain about greedy doctors — there certainly are some — but it is long-term health care that bankrupts the elderly. Few patients deplete all their assets paying doctors' and hospital bills. However, rarely will Medicare cover nursing home care. Medicaid (MediCal in California), the program for the poor, will pay for nursing home care but only after you have exhausted your assets.

Medicare was enacted in 1966 and because it covers virtually anyone over 65, few over this age-group are without health insurance.

```
SIMPLIFIED OVERVIEW OF MEDICARE
           COVERAGE

    Part A                    Part B

Hospital Expenses         Doctors fees
Home Care                 Outpatient Surgery
Hospice Care              Outpatient X-rays
Skilled Nursing Care      Outpatient lab work
                          Physical Therapy
                          Speech Therapy
                          Medical Supplies
                          Hospice Care
                          Home Care
```

Figure 2-1

While it has been largely successful, it has outstripped its predicted expenses. In 1966, economists predicted Medicare would cost 8 billion dollars annually by 1990, even after adjusted for inflation. The actual cost was 90 billion dollars.

Medicare is one of the most complex social programs ever enacted. Neither the patients, doctors, politicians nor administrators understand it completely. What follows is a simplified explanation of Medicare. A more detailed discussion of the nuances of Medicare is found in *Social Security, Medicare and Pensions* by Joseph L. Matthews from Nolo Press. Other than some requisite doctor-bashing, this book explains the complex subject in as simple a fashion as possible.

Medicare does not provide full health insurance coverage and rarely provides for nursing home care. It is divided into two parts, Part A and Part B (Figure 2-1). In most cases, those who are 65 are automatically eligible for Part A. Those who retire earlier and those who opt for social security at age 62 are not eligible for Medicare until they are age 65. People who are disabled for a total of 24 months can receive Medicare at any age. The law defining a disability is complex and draconian. An individual with kidney failure requiring dialysis is automatically eligible for Medicare, but other ailments are not as clear-

SUMMARY OF MEDICARE PART A

How hospital bills are paid for a given illness:
First 60 days..... Full coverage after $628 (1991) deductible
61-90 days......... Patient pays $157 (1991) per day. The remainder is
paid by Medicare
91 to 150 days .. Patient pays $314 (1991) per day and Medicare
covers the remainder. This is for a total of 60 days per lifetime.
After 150 days.. No coverage

Skilled-Nursing-Home Care (e.g. dressings, injections etc.):*
First 20 days........ Full coverage
21 to 100 days...... Patient pays $78.50 (1991) a day. The remainder is
paid by Medicare up to $6,280 per illness.
After 100 days..... No coverage
Hospice Care...... Full coverage if requirements are met

Unskilled-Nursing-Home Care (feeding, bathing etc.) - No coverage

Home-health care........ 100% coverage if requirements are met:
(i.e. unable to leave the house, home care ordered by your doctor, periodic nursing care, speech therapy and physical therapy)

*must be discharged from a hospital to qualify

Figure 2-2

cut. Individuals denied Medicare disability have the right to appeal
and reversals occur in 50% of cases.

Part A covers inpatient hospital expenses, some skilled-nursing
care, home care and hospice care and has an inpatient deductible of
$628 (1991). Part B is optional and covers doctor expenses, outpatient
hospital and laboratory charges, home-health care, X-rays, physical
and speech therapy, some medications and a few medical supplies.
Those who opt for Part B have $29.90 (1991) deducted from their social
security check every month.

```
┌─────────────────────────────────────────────────────────┐
│                                                         │
│      SIMPLIFIED SUMMARY OF MEDICARE PART B              │
│                                                         │
│   Doctors' Bills.........................  80% of approved amount*    │
│   Outpatient Hospital Bills .......  80% of approved amount     │
│   Outpatient Medical Services ..  80% of approved amount     │
│   Home-health care....................  100% of approved amount    │
│   Hospice Care .........................  100% of approved amount    │
│                                                         │
│      *after $100 deductible                            │
│                                                         │
└─────────────────────────────────────────────────────────┘
```

Figure 2-3

Part B has an annual deductible of $100 (1991) and covers 80% of "approved charges" (Figure 2-1). Medicare Part A covers the expenses of the first 60 days of hospitalization per given illness, but only a portion thereafter (Figure 2-2). It does not pay for help with the activities of daily living (ADL's in the bureaucratic vernacular) – dressing, walking, bathing, using the bathroom and meals. This "custodial care" is often more important to the elderly than medical care. "Skilled care" is covered and includes dressing changes, administering intravenous antibiotics, and caring for catheters. If you find the above distinctions confusing and illogical, you are not alone.

Part B (Figure 2-3) only pays 80% of the approved charges whether it is for a doctor bill or for a treatment. The patient has the option of going to a physician who either does or does not take "assignment." A doctor who takes assignment agrees to accept the government's reimbursement. Medicare will then pay 80% of the assigned amount and the patient or the patient's co-insurance is responsible for the difference. If this sounds confusing, that's because it is. For example, assume a patient has met his $100 deductible and goes to a doctor who charges $100 for her services. If this doctor accepts assignment, she will be reimbursed $80 by the government. The patient's insurance company or the patient himself is then responsible for the remaining $20. Incidentally, it is illegal for doctors not to charge for the 20% owed to them. This is to discourage fraud by having doctors bill the government for large amounts of money without charging the patient anything. All Medicare recipients receive a booklet that lists the names of doctors in their area that accept assignment.

Doctors who do not accept assignment are also limited in the amount of money they can charge patients if they are to be partially paid by Medicare. These are called MAAC's (maximally allowable charges) and all doctors who are registered with Medicare but who do not accept assignment receive a profile of what they are permitted to charge. Co-insurance may or may not pick up this difference. For example, return to the same patient in the previous paragraph. In this instance, the doctor does not accept assignment and charges her MAAC of $125. The government reimburses her $75 (this is less than for those who take assignment) and the patient is then responsible for $50. Some insurance policies may pay all $50, others may pay only $20 and others may pay nothing at all. Trying to make sense of how insurance companies pay health care bills is a waste of time. It frequently depends upon the mood of the claims adjustor rather than what the policy specifies. Getting reimbursed is mostly a function of the patient's drive and persistence.

Those on Medicare have the option of obtaining private supplemental insurance called Medigap. There are many different policies and they may or may not have deductibles. For example, a policy may or may not cover the $628 (1991) deductible of Part A but leave you protected for hospital expenses incurred over Medicare's 90-day hospitalization limit. Some policies may only cover the assigned-doctors bills so that if your doctor does not take assignment, you are responsible for the difference. Usually only one insurance policy is necessary. Do not be enticed into buying several. Overlapping supplemental insurance policies are commonly sold to the elderly. Also, remember the main rule in purchasing any insurance policy: if it sounds too good to be true, it probably is.

Medicaid was designed to take care of the poor. In some states such as Connecticut, Medicaid will pay the 20% of the assigned amount not covered by Medicare Part B and in other states such as New York, it will not. Medicaid is much more relevant in the discussion of long-term health care.

LONG-TERM HEALTH CARE

The expense of long-term health care is the main fear of the elderly today. Poor planning can divide a close family by the animosity created from the dissipation of a loved one's estate. Discussions on whether to proceed with aggressive treatment are often based on financial as well as medical considerations. Medicare will not pay for long-term health care except under specific circumstances and then only for a limited period. I am sorry to keep repeating this but if you remember one fact from this chapter, make sure it is this one.

Skilled-nursing-home care benefits cover the first 20 days. For the next 80 days, you must pay $78.50 (1991) a day. After that, you are on your own. If you are admitted to a nursing home for custodial care — as most patients are — nothing is covered. Few private health-care plans cover long-term health care and many middle-class and upper middle-class Americans have had their life savings decimated by these expenses. However, both Part A and Part B will pay for home care and hospice care if certain requirements are met.

There are several ways of providing yourself with long-term care:

1. Hiring help to care for you at home.
2. Entering a retirement community
3. Living with a family member
4. Entering a nursing home
5. Entering a hospice when your condition is terminal

Staying In Your Home

Most people become attached to their homes and prefer to remain there when ill. The problem is that houses can be expensive to maintain even if the mortgage is paid. Taxes keep increasing and routine chores such as lawn maintenance, snow shovelling, house cleaning and minor repairs can become herculean tasks. Houses purchased during youth and middle age may become an obstacle course for the elderly because of steep stairs, sloped driveways, and narrow bathrooms. Again, those with significant financial resources can modify their houses by installing ramps, grab bars, additional bathrooms, chairlifts or elevators.

Many communities have services such as Meals-on-Wheels, which delivers food to the elderly at reduced costs. Low-cost transportation services may be available. Public and private home-service agencies provide homemakers that can help with domestic chores for $5 to $15 an hour. Those who have trouble bathing and using the bathroom can hire home-health aids but they are more expensive, typically $10-$25 an hour — depending on the level of care. Only those with considerable financial reserves can afford this type of care.

Medicare Part A or B will pay for part-time skilled-nursing care at home and Part B will pay for physical therapy and speech therapy at home. You must be sick enough so that you cannot leave your home, to qualify. Unlike skilled-nursing care in the nursing home, you do not have to be discharged from a hospital to qualify. All you need is a statement from your doctor. Most areas have home-health-care agencies that participate in Medicare and the service is frequently under-utilized. Many elderly are unfairly denied this benefit and this may be legally challenged. There is a high ruling-rate in favor of the patient.

Trading down to a smaller but more convenient home or a condo can make life easier without foregoing autonomy. It may also be to your financial advantage because you can take the one-time exclusion allowed for those over 55 years old. You are permitted to keep up to $125,000 profit from the sale of your house without paying the federal capital gains tax.

For example, if you sell your house for a profit of $220,000 and purchase a condo or another house for $100,000 over the purchase price of your initial house, the $120,000 difference is yours without taxes. On the other hand, if the profit on this transaction was $160,000, you could keep $125,000 tax-free, but would have to pay the capital gains tax on the remaining $35,000.

Entering a retirement community

Another option is to enter an elder-care community. There are a variety of alternatives ranging from communities with minimal assistance to those with round-the-clock nursing care. Some communities will jettison you if you become incapacitated while others promise to care for you. The latter can be expensive, requiring anywhere from $20,000 to $250,000 up-front, followed by a monthly maintenance fee.

Some of these facilities are excellent but others were built in the speculative frenzy of the 1980's and may renege on their promises. The owners have the "I'll cross that bridge when I come to it" attitude and if they encounter financial difficulties, they simply raise fees and cut services. Your only recourse is to sue and even if you win, the owner's money is probably ensconced in the Cayman Islands and the only thing you end up with is legal bills. While recent laws have been passed to prevent abuses, often it is better to enter a community with high monthly fees but a minimal down payment. If the community does not meet your standards or decreases services, you simply move.

Living with your children

The media like to portray baby boomers as self-centered and materialistic. Yet most of these boomers look after their parents when necessary. Sixty percent of elderly adults move in with their children.

Returning to live with your children is a mixed blessing. Old animosities that have been buried for years may resurface. Your child's spouse may wonder why his parents were not treated in such a favorable fashion. If one sibling bears more responsibility than others, he may feel that he deserves a larger share of your estate. The key is to ascertain the reasonable expectations of you and your children with regard to financial and emotional support prior to moving. For example, building an addition to your child's house can have beneficial tax benefits, but your other children may perceive this investment as an unfair disbursement of your estate. Overall though, with the use of adult day-care and home-health care, living with your children is most often a comfortable way to spend your final years.

Entering a nursing home

Nonetheless, even with the best intentions, a significant portion of the elderly require nursing home care – 25% of those over 65 and 50% of those 90 and over. Nursing homes vary from outstanding to grossly negligent. It is a good idea to put your name on the list of a reputable nursing home before you become incapacitated. Being placed in a nursing home often causes tremendous family anxiety and guilt. It shouldn't, because in most cases, there is no choice. A good source of information about nursing homes is:

National Citizens' Coalition for Nursing Home Reform
1424 16 St. NW, Suite L2
Washington, DC 20036
202-797-0657

Nursing home care can cost anywhere from $20,000 to $80,000 a year depending upon the level of care and the cost of living in the home's locale. Sixty-five percent of nursing home patients deplete their assets after only 13 weeks of care and the average nursing home stay is three years. Medicaid was initially proposed to care for poor people under 65. However, with the increased necessity of long-term health care, many middle-class Americans have been forced to deplete all their assets in order to obtain Medicaid coverage for long-term care. As a matter of fact, 41% of nursing home bills are paid by Medicaid and in New York state, 45% of the Medicaid bill is for long-term care. Medicaid is partially state and partially federally funded, thus there is considerable variation from state to state. While the rules have changed recently so that couples do not have to become destitute prior to Medicaid eligibility, they are quite restrictive and infinitely complex. It is paramount that those planning for their long-term care consult both a lawyer and an accountant who are well-versed in this area.

Some broad concepts do apply. If you are single or both you and your spouse require long-term care simultaneously, you are required to liquidate your assets including the sale of your house until you each have a net worth of $1,600 (this varies from state to state), the approximate cost of an inexpensive funeral. Only then are you eligible for Medicaid. On the other hand, if only one spouse is being institutionalized, some assets, like a house (if the other spouse still lives there) and some types of annuities and trusts, are protected. A house is also protected if a disabled child lives there, or if a sibling or child has lived there for a period of time and has equity interest in the house.

You are not permitted to transfer your assets for thirty months prior to eligibility for Medicaid. If you sell your assets, the government will check to see if the transaction is appropriate. For example, if you sell your $175,000 house for $35,000 to your son, you could be accused of improper transfer and therefore not eligible for Medicaid for a period of time. Again, these rules vary from state to state and are constantly changing so expert advice is imperative. In Connecticut, for example, a single person who enters a nursing home does not have to sell his house to pay for long-term care if a doctor certifies that he will be able to return to his home within nine months. Obviously, no doctor can accurately predict this, so it is possible that a single person could lose his house to pay for long-term care.

A recent change, effective July 30, 1989 permits a spouse who stays at her home to keep her house and receive a reasonable stipend from her husband's income even while Medicaid pays for her husband's long-term health care. Factors such as mortgages, taxes, food expenses, insurance and utilities are considered. An assessment is done by the local Medicaid agency and—if necessary—the judiciary. Unfortunately, federal laws sometimes limit this stipend so as not to exceed $1,500 a month, which is inadequate in some parts of the country. On the other hand, if the spouse has assets or income of her own, these must be considered. Thus when the husband enters the nursing home, the assets of both are assessed and considered. The value of their house is not included in this assessment.

The at-home spouse is permitted to keep half the total assets up to $66,480 (1991 - adjusted annually for inflation). If the total assets are less than $24,000, the spouse can keep at least $13,296 (1991); even, for instance, if the assets total only $14,000. The husband's share of this assessment must then be spent until it is reduced to $1,600 (this varies from state to state) and then Medicaid will pay for his care. A common misconception is that the husband's share must be spent only on nursing home care. Actually, it can be spent by the at-home spouse for living expenses such as food, clothing and home improvements.

For example, an elderly man may need to enter a nursing home but his wife is healthy. They purchased their house for $30,000 but now it is worth $250,000. They have no mortgage but she requires $450 a month to maintain the house and $900 a month for living expenses. He receives $400 in Social Security and she receives $300. They have combined assets of $80,000 in stocks and bonds. If the wife prefers to remain in their house, it can not be included in the assessment by Medicaid. Generally, their $80,000 will be split in half and she can keep

$40,000. The husbands $40,000 share can be spent for his long-term care but it may also be used to fix the roof or finish the basement. When this fund is depleted to $1,600, Medicaid will pay for his long-term care. Since she requires about $1,350 a month in living expenses, she is permitted to keep her and her husband's social security allocation. After her husband has passed away she may need to enter a nursing home too. She must then spend down all of her remaining assets to qualify for Medicaid. This includes selling her house unless a doctor states she will return to her home within nine months (in Connecticut). The proceeds from the sale are used to pay her nursing home bills until she qualifies for Medicaid. While this example is oversimplified, it typifies the issues that must be considered when planning long-term care.

Some "clever" financial planners recommend buying a long-term health-insurance policy that pays for only 30 months. This way you are covered for the period required before you can legally transfer all your assets. While this appears to be expedient, it could prove devastating in terms of gift and estate tax consequences. If enough people do it, the government may simply increase the 30-month time period.

Often patients do not anticipate when they will enter a nursing home. The usual scenario involves a parent who is living with his children and is admitted to the hospital for a disease such as pneumonia. Hospitals are paid by Medicare by a system called DRG's (Diagnostic Related Groups) whereby the hospital is paid for a specified number of days depending on the disease. In this case, let's say it is 10 days. If the hospital can discharge the patient before 10 days, it makes a profit but if the recovery period is longer, the hospital loses money. What often happens, though, is the patient's pneumonia is cured but he refuses to go home or the overwhelmed family refuses to accept him. It is illegal for the hospital to discharge him onto the street. Now the hospital is in a position where it has a bed occupied that is not generating revenue.

This gives the hospital administrator ulcers and he quickly dispatches a social worker to find a bed for the patient in a nursing home. The nursing home is happy to take the patient if he spends down his assets. This causes considerable consternation within the family as they have had no time to prepare. Remember, the patient is not eligible for Medicaid if he has transferred his assets within the last 30 months.

37

If he refuses to go to the nursing home, the hospital is free to bill him for each day he stays over 10 days. This can be $700 dollars a day. Unlike doctors, who are poor at collecting delinquent accounts, hospitals hire batteries of lawyers who have remarkable talents when it comes to collecting bills. They will freeze his bank accounts and put a lien on his house. If he has recently transferred assets, they will accuse him of fraud. Thus it is imperative that plans for long-term care be made well in advance.

Even if you are clever enough to transfer your assets to qualify for Medicaid, you may regret it. Medicaid simply does not pay nursing homes enough money to break even, so the nursing homes are constantly plotting to get Medicaid patients out of their facilities and replace them with paying patients. Nursing homes are prohibited from discharging you because you are on Medicaid, but what happens if you become ill and have to be placed in the hospital. This is a very common scenario. In Connecticut, the nursing home has the right to fill your bed if you are not back in 14 days, but in Massachusetts, the period is only 10 days. In other states, the time period is even shorter.

For example, while in a nursing home you have a bad heart attack requiring protracted hospitalization. When it's time to return to the nursing home, your bed is gone. The hospital administrator's ulcer starts acting up again. He disperses battalions of social workers to comb the state and find you a bed. He unleashes utilization review, a government-mandated cost-control department in all hospitals, on your attending physician. Your doctor must then start ordering tests and create a new diagnosis for you to justify your continued stay or Medicare will not pay your hospital bill. When a bed is eventually found, it may be in a substandard facility that is willing to take a Medicaid patient.

Another problem with transferring assets, especially your house, is they may end up in the hands of others. For example, you give your house to your daughter who agrees to allow you to stay there for the rest of your life. However, she gets divorced and after an ugly legal battle, your son-in-law—whom you never liked anyway—gets the house. You're soon out on the street. One of my patients transferred her house to her married son. He was tragically killed in an accident and the house passed to his spouse. Everything was fine until her daughter-in-law remarried, at which point she was drop kicked out of her own house. In another instance, a house that an elderly woman had given to her son was used as collateral for a business loan. When the business went bankrupt, the bank seized the house. These are common occurrences that happen to ordinary people all the time. Keep them in mind when you are transferring your assets.

Thus, if you have the financial resources to pay for your own long-term care, you will always have some control over your destiny. Clever plans that enable you to protect your estate from taxes and long-term health-care bills may nevertheless result in substandard and undignified care, or the loss of your assets due to contingencies you could not possibly have foreseen.

* * *

Recently, insurance policies are becoming the vogue to cover long-term care. They are expensive and replete with loopholes and pitfalls. Many people have paid into these policies for years only to discover that their insurance company's doctor must approve their nursing home admission, that the coverage did not adjust for inflation and does not come close to covering nursing home costs, or that the insurance company has gone belly-up.

Thus, the wealthy may want to forgo insurance because they can pay for long-term care if necessary. Those with few assets may not find it prudent to pay large premiums since Medicaid offers them a safety-net. It is those with an intermediate net worth, between $200,000 and $800,000, who might consider obtaining a policy.

It is possible to obtain these policies at a young age, even before age 50. At this age, the cost is about $250 a year and is fixed for the duration of the policy. Naturally, like life insurance, the rate increases depending upon the age you purchase the policy. A 70-year-old man can expect to pay $1,500 a year and and 80-year-old man, $4,500. There are a variety of pitfalls that must be avoided when purchasing this type of insurance:

1. Make sure the insurance company cannot cancel the policy if your health status changes. Also make sure that pre-existing conditions, such as Alzheimer's or Parkinson's (diseases in which the patient can live for a long time), are not excluded from coverage.

2. Make sure there is no fine print that permits the insurance company to arbitrarily raise premiums.

3. There should be no insurance company physician who can decide whether you belong in a nursing home. It should be your decision when you can no longer care for yourself.

4. You should not have to be admitted to a hospital before being placed in the nursing home.

5. If you are fortunate enough to know the geographical locale of your future nursing home, make sure the policy pays enough to cover the anticipated costs. For example, if the cost is $100 a day, this should be your amount of coverage. If you are uncertain, make sure that it is at least $90 a day and that this will be adjusted annually for inflation (even this may be inadequate as health care costs have been increasing at a much more rapid rate than inflation). This should be calculated in a compounded fashion or else when you need the policy, it will not cover your expenses.

6. It should also cover home care or hospice care. Remember, the best place to spend you final years is in your home. However, keep in mind that home care is more expensive than nursing home care and the daily allowance of your policy may be inadequate, forcing you to use your assets.

7. Make sure the policy not only pays for skilled-nursing care but also for custodial care.

8. There should be no limits on the benefit period. Do not be assuaged if a pushy salesman informs you that the average nursing home stay is only six months. Those who are discharged eventually have to reenter so that on the average, a person who enters a nursing home can expect to spend three years of his life there.

If you find the above recommendations too overwhelming, you may want to avoid purchasing long-term-care insurance. With the population aging, there may be clamor for government-backed financing for long-term care and you may have spent a lot of money for nothing. It is also possible that when today's youngsters get the bill for the baby boomer's long-term care, euthanasia will be legalized in short order. There is also a movement to allow the dying to receive their life insurance premiums to pay for their health care, the so-called accelerated-death benefit. Anyone under 65 purchasing long-term health insurance must understand that it will be a completely different world by the time they require care.

A free guide, The Consumer's Guide to Long-Term Care, is available from:

The Health Insurance Association of America
1025 Connecticut Ave. NW
Washington, DC 20036

Hospice Care

Hospices are dedicated to providing pain control and symptom management in the terminally ill and they have moved into the mainstream of patient care. A hospice may be a physical building or an organization dedicated to providing home care for the dying. Medicare, Medicaid, Blue Cross/Blue Shield and most health insurance policies cover hospice care. Hospices are not overly expensive and are run by dedicated professionals who are committed to helping the dying. The main problem is that not enough doctors and patients use them. Medicare will pay for hospice care if a physician states the following:

1. The patient has a poor chance of living over six months.
2. No known treatment is effective.
3. The patient has appointed a health care proxy.

The patient must agree not to accept treatment for conditions other than symptom relief and must enrol in a Medicare-certified hospice program. These are listed in the Yellow Pages. Until recently, Medicare only paid 210 days of hospice care, but now coverage has been extended to pay indefinitely. Once you have made the decision to enter a hospice, Medicare limits your hospital coverage. However, you may opt to leave hospice coverage and return to full Medicare coverage. While in the hospice program, your doctor bills are still covered for unrelated conditions, the fees for medications are small and there are no deductibles. Dying patients are well-advised to consider hospice care.

PLANNING FOR ESTATE TAXES

With an increasing budget deficit, the government will be searching for ways to raise revenue without raising the public ire. One of the best ways is by increasing inheritance taxes. This arcane type of law is practiced by few lawyers and understood by even fewer. It is estimated that today's senior citizens have assets exceeding 8 trillion dollars and the government is licking its chops. All politicians know that supporting a tax increase on wages can shorten their careers but few elections turn on a candidate's position on inheritance taxes. In Scott Turow's novel *The Burden of Proof*, the major character, Alejendro Stern, proudly notes that his wife's $8,000,000 estate has no taxes due after her death. This may be the province of fiction, but intelligent planning can result in massive savings in estate taxes.

Thus, everyone must have their estate in order to avoid unexpected tax bills. Federal tax on estates does not begin until the estate exceeds $600,000 in value. While many feel that such a large amount ensures their safety from worry, many families are surprised with large tax bills because their estates are bigger than they realized. Owning two homes is not uncommon for senior citizens. Life insurance (it is often taxable in spite of what insurance salesmen tell you), annuities, and family businesses are also included in one's estate. Also state taxes usually are assessed on estates less than $600,000. For example, in Connecticut, state taxes are due on estates over $50,000 at a rate starting at 4.29%. If you own houses in two states, the laws of each state must be considered. Also, many people think that they can simply transfer large amounts of money to a spouse tax-free. While this is true, what happens when the spouse dies? For example, if a wife dies and her husband is now the sole owner of a $800,000 estate, when he dies,

$200,000 will be taxed. However, if she had left $200,000 to her children and the remaining $600,000 to her husband, the tax is avoided.

There are other ways to avoid these taxes. Gifts of up to $10,000 may be dispersed annually. Thus, a married couple may give $20,000 to each of their children and grandchildren. Trusts can be established that avoid taxes. Decisions on whether or not to avoid treatment are often much easier when one has peace of mind knowing that the estate one has labored to acquire will not be seized by the government.

PLANNING FOR THE DISBURSEMENT OF YOUR ESTATE

There is little sense in going through the arcane complexities of avoiding estate taxes and high long-term health care bills unless you go through the inconvenience and expense of obtaining and updating a will. Not only does this make life easier for your heirs, it can also prevent an acrimonious battle. Ralph Waldo Emerson put it best when he stated, "When it comes to dividing an estate, even the most polite of men quarrel."

After you die, your estate is taken through a procedure called probate, the legal process of validating your will — if you have one — and disbursing your estate. This can take months if you are among the 65% of people who die intestate, that is, without a will. The estate cannot be inherited unless all taxes are paid. This may force your family to sell your house in a weak market for less than its value or even take out a large loan if your estate has inadequate liquid assets. Having a current will and planning ahead makes life easier for everyone.

Avoid the temptation to use generic or computer-software-generated wills. Legal technicalities can cause them to be thrown out in court. Even if you have no ostensible heirs, you should have a will. Many people are under the impression that if they die without obvious heirs, the estate goes to the government. This isn't true. It goes to your parents. If they are dead, it goes to their siblings. If they are dead, it goes to their siblings' children (your cousins). This is why you read in the paper every so often that someone inherited money from a obscure relative.

HAVING OTHERS HANDLE YOUR FINANCIAL AFFAIRS IF
YOU BECOME INCAPACITATED

If you have not set up a mechanism for others to tend to your affairs should you become incompetent, the judicial system will do it for you. ˜he mechanism is called guardianship or conservatorship. This is the most common and most restrictive and intrusive form of intervention. The court appoints a third party (the guardian or conservator) to assume the affairs of a person (the ward) when the court finds him to be incompetent or incapacitated. This may be a family member, friend, attorney or a public guardian. With guardianship, the ward loses many fundamental rights. Although these vary from state to state – they may include the right to enter into contracts, decide where to live (e.g. your home versus a nursing home), to hold a driver's license (a major fear of older Americans), and to manage one's own assets and affairs. Thus, older Americans must not only plan for their death but also for the possibility of functional impairment.

If you have the desire to prevent this problem you have a variety of options depending upon the laws of your state. These include:

> Power of Attorney
> Durable Power of Attorney
> Representative Payee
> Joint Ownership
> Living Trust

Power of Attorney. This gives someone else the legal right to manage your affairs. It is a comprehensive document that confers to your designated agent the power to manage your affairs which may include financial as well as health, such as consenting to surgery. Please look at Connecticut's power of attorney form (Figure 2-4). This is a powerful document and lawyers facetiously refer to it as a "license to steal." However, it becomes inactive once you become incapacitated.

Durable Power of Attorney. In this case, your designated agent can act on your behalf even after you become incapacitated. In Connecticut, the statement with the asterisk at the bottom of the document must be included. The designated agent may be a family member but you

44

CONNECTICUT'S SHORT FORM FOR POWER OF ATTORNEY

Know all Men by these presents, which are intended to constitute a General Power of Attorney pursuant to Connecticut Statutory Short Form Power of Attorney Act: That I_____do hereby appoint_____ my attorney(s)-in-fact to act:
(a)First: in my name, place and stead in any way which I myself could do, if I were personally present, with respect to the following matters as each of them is defined in the Connecticut Statutory Short Form Power of Attorney Act to the extent that I am permitted by law to act through an agent: (Strike out and initial in the opposite box any one or more of the subdivisions as to which the principal does NOT desire to give the agent authority. Such elimination of any one or more subdivisions (A) to (L), inclusive, shall automatically constitute an elimination also of subdivision (M).)

To strike out any subdivisions the principal must draw a line through the text of that subdivision AND write his initials in the box opposite.

(A) real estate transactions;   [ ]
(B) chattel and goods transactions;   [ ]
(C) bond, share and commodity transactions;   [ ]
(D) banking transactions;   [ ]
(E) business operating transactions;   [ ]
(F) insurance transactions;   [ ]
(G) estate transactions;   [ ]
(H) claims and litigation;   [ ]
(I) personal relationships and affairs;   [ ]
(J) benefits from military service;   [ ]
(K) records, reports and statements;   [ ]
(L) health care decisions;   [ ]
(M) all other matters;   [ ]

This power or attorney shall not be affected by the subsequent disability or incompetence of the principal*

*the inclusion of this statement makes this a durable power of attorney. If not included, the document is void if the principal becomes incapacitated. If "(L) health care decisions" is initialed, then this document may also serve as a health care proxy.

Figure 2-4

45

may designate a close friend or a trusted lawyer who has no financial interest in your estate and is unencumbered by family politics. In Connecticut, this document may be used as a health care proxy, but other states have a specific document.

Representative Payee. This is someone appointed by a government agency such as the Social Security Administration or a state pension board who oversees the money you receive from that agency. This person can only disperse funds from said agency.

Living Trust. This is when you transfer your assets to a separate entity (the trust) that is managed by another person you designate (the trustee) while you are still alive. When you die, the trust avoids probate so that a trust can substitute partially for a will. However, there are still tax consequences that must be considered. Also, if a trust is abused, it is very difficult to extricate the trustee from the agreement.

Joint Ownership. This is when you give another individual(s) access to your money or possessions. For example, you may put your daughter's name on the deed to your house so that it is transferred to her automatically when you die. Many elderly also give a child joint ownership of a bank account for the sake of convenience. The account may be structured so that the permission of both of you is required to withdraw money. This is fine as long as you are mentally competent, but what happens if you are not. This contingency can be circumvented by structuring the account so that either you or your child can withdraw money without permission of the other, but the potential for abuse is obvious. Other problems may also arise. Joint ownership can become a headache if you are trying to qualify for Medicaid to fund your nursing home care. It also can cause problems with gift and estate taxes. Family feuds may begin if the joint owner of your account or house refuses to share it with the rest of your family when you pass away. Often a child who is the joint owner of a house will view it as payment for performing the lion's share of the work in the care of elderly parents. Her siblings may not agree.

SUMMARY

Everyone must assess financial factors when confronting a terminal illness. Patients rarely become insolvent due to doctor and hospital bills because of the protection of Medicare. It is long-term health care that results in insolvency because Medicaid only pays for it after you have depleted all your assets. You can avoid these expenses by transferring assets to heirs well in advance of the anticipated need for long-term care. However, this results in the loss of control of your affairs. A hospice or your own house is the best place to spend your final days, but sometimes it is impossible to avoid a nursing home. Consider money spent on competent financial and legal advice as a sound investment. If a doctor says this, you know it must be true.

Chapter 3

LEGAL ASPECTS OF REFUSING TREATMENT: WHAT RIGHTS YOU HAVE AND WHAT RIGHTS YOU DON'T HAVE

The legal aspects regarding treatment and the termination of treatment are changing on a daily basis and vary widely from state to state (refer to Appendix 2 for the the laws of each state). Gradually, a consensus is evolving in our judicial and legislative bodies that life-prolonging treatment in terminal patients is fruitless and that it is also reasonable to withdraw treatment in these cases. Remember, you already possess the fundamental right to have control of your death — the right to refuse treatment. If you are incapacitated and unable to exercise that right, there are two ways to make your wishes known: living wills (advanced directives) and health care proxies (Figure 3-1). Sometimes these overlap.

All the legal documents in the world cannot supercede the main issue in terminal-patient care — trust. If you trust your doctor to look after your best interests and trust your family to handle your affairs when you are incapacitated, the protection afforded by living wills and health care proxies becomes a secondary issue. A good physician will answer questions regarding prognosis and whether continued treatment will be beneficial or futile. Ask your doctor what he would do if his mother had the same condition. If your doctor will not answer

```
┌─────────────────────────────────────────────────────────────┐
│                                                               │
│       LEGAL DOCUMENTS REGARDING TREATMENT                     │
│                                                               │
│     Living Will - states what treatment you want to refuse    │
│     Health Care Proxy - an individual you designate to make   │
│           your health care decisions if you are incapacitated │
│                                                               │
│                                                               │
└─────────────────────────────────────────────────────────────┘
```

Figure 3-1

questions to your satisfaction, find one who will, but remember, your doctor does not have a crystal ball.

Your doctor must also trust you. If he is afraid that your family is going to sue him or report him to the State Board of Health for not exhausting all therapeutic options when your condition is terminal, he will protect his interests and not yours. Recent legislation has established a National Practitioner's Data Bank to register complaints and malpractice actions against doctors. While it has the laudable goals of protecting the public from incompetent doctors, it is making some doctors paranoid. A doctor who has his name filed in the Data Bank for an incident that is beyond his control can lose his hospital privileges and therefore his livelihood.

LIVING WILLS

A living will is a legal statement that rejects in advance heroic medical treatment if the patient becomes terminally ill. Forty-eight states and the District of Columbia recognize living wills and some states have had them for 25 years. Legal requirements vary from state to state and most states do not respect the living wills of other states. Thus if you are visiting Texas, your living will from Colorado has no clout.

Living wills are far from a panacea. The living will used in Connecticut is shown in Figure 3-2. Please read it carefully. This is

SAMPLE OF THE LIVING WILL FROM THE STATE OF CONNECTICUT

TO WHOM IT MAY CONCERN, INCLUDING MY FAMILY, MY PHYSICIAN, MY CLERGYMAN AND MY LAWYER

If the time comes when I am incapacitated to the point where I can no longer actively take part in decisions for my own life and am unable to direct my physician as to my own medical care, I wish this statement to stand as a testament of my wishes. I request that, if my condition is deemed terminal or if I am determined to be permanently unconscious, I be allowed to die and not be kept alive through life support systems. By terminal condition, I mean that I have an incurable or irreversible medical condition which without the administration of life support systems will, in the opinion of my attending physician, result in death within a relatively short time. By permanently unconscious, I mean that I am in a permanent coma or persistent vegetative state which is an irreversible condition in which I am at no time aware of myself or the environment and show no behavioral response to the environment. The life support systems which I do not want included, but are not limited to, are artificial respiration, cardiopulmonary resuscitation and artificial means of providing nutrition and hydration. I direct that medication be liberally administered to me to alleviate pain even though it may hasten the moment of my death. I do not intend any direct taking of my life, but only that my dying not be unreasonably prolonged. This request is made, after careful reflection, while I am of sound mind.

Signature _____

Date _____   Witness _____

Figure 3-2

50

one of the most progressive in the country because the terms "terminal condition" and "persistent vegetative state" are defined. Not all states give the patient this luxury. In some states, a persistent vegetative state is not considered a terminal condition because the patient can survive for decades. The concept of "sound mind" will probably be debated by the legal profession for eternity. Terminal patients are often confused because of their debilitated state or side effects of medications. Connecticut's living will considers feeding tubes to be a "life support system," along with respirators and CPR. In other states, a feeding tube is not included in this category and thus could be inserted against your will or the wishes of your family.

Many a surprised family has found a living will to be ineffective. In most states, a doctor can override a living will without penalty. For instance, you have chest pain and call an ambulance. In the emergency room, you lose consciousness and are intubated and placed on a respirator. Even if you have suffered irreversible brain damage, a doctor will be reluctant to remove the respirator and end your life simply on the strength of a piece of paper. Physicians are more comfortable dealing either with a dying but coherent patient or a health care proxy where a relationship based on frank discussions and mutual trust can be established.

While living wills do have deficiencies, they at least alert your doctor to the fact that you wish to have control over your death. Your doctor may be reluctant to make decisions without consulting you or your family. One final caveat. Make sure a copy of your living will is in your doctor's chart. Make certain that your family knows where your copy is kept and that they have several copies themselves.

HEALTH CARE PROXY

A health care proxy allows another individual to make decisions for you in case you are incapacitated. In some states, it is incorporated in the living will. In others, it may be an extension of durable power of attorney as discussed in the previous chapter. All states have durable power of attorney which allow others to take over the financial affairs of incompetent individuals. Only recently has this been extrapolated to health care decisions. On the opposite page is the health care proxy form used in the state of New York (Figure 3-3).

A recent case in New York exemplifies the advantage of a health care proxy. An AIDS patient was admitted to a hospital with a brain infection that rendered him incoherent. The patient's companion showed the doctor the patient's living will. The doctor, noting the patient had an infection that was potentially reversible with antibiotics, treated him anyway. The patient died but the case went to court and the doctor was exonerated. It was reasoned that although the patient had a terminal disease, his infection was theoretically curable. Now if the patient had made his companion his health care proxy, his companion would have had legal stature and could have refused treatment. Thus health care proxies can step in when living wills are inadequate. If your family is faced with health care decisions when you are incompetent, it is much easier if one family member is designated as your health care proxy. This should be an individual who knows and understands your philosophy about your life being prolonged by artificial life-support systems.

Health care proxies are not recognized in every state and many states place restrictions on the treatments that can be refused. Note that in New York, a health care proxy cannot prevent a feeding tube from being placed unless it is specifically stated in the document. Another problem with a health care proxy is that a doctor may be reluctant to let a patient die if the family disagrees on the best course of action, even though from a legal point of view, one person has the power to make the decision. Family dynamics are such that even if the majority of family members feel a loved one should be allowed to die peacefully, they will acquiesce to one family member who wants to continue with aggressive and futile care. Remember, the doctor does not want to be sued, even if the law is on his side because it makes his life miserable. Thus, if some relative arrives at your bedside from the hinterlands and insists on a full-court press, your doctor may acquiesce to this relative's wishes, even if his view is a minority in the family.

HEALTH CARE PROXY FOR THE STATE OF NEW YORK

I _____, hereby appoint
_____as my health care agent to
make any and all health care decisions for me, except to the extent that
I state otherwise. This proxy shall take effect when and if I become
unable to make my own health care decisions. I direct my agent to
make health care decisions in accord with my wishes and limitations as
stated below or as he or she otherwise knows.

_____

_____ (THE PATIENT WRITES HERE
WHAT TREATMENT SHE DOES NOT DESIRE SUCH AS A
FEEDING TUBE)

Name of substitute or fill-in agent if the person I appoint above
is unable, unwilling or unavailable to act as my health care
agent. _____
Unless I revoke it, this proxy shall remain in effect indefinitely, or
until the date or conditions stated here: _____

Signature _____

Date _____   Witness _____

Figure 3-3

WITHDRAWING TREATMENT

Exercising your right to refuse treatment, living wills and health care proxies are helpful if you have a terminal disease, but what if you and your doctor are unsure whether treatment with a respirator or feeding tube will help. For example, a scenario arises in which after an operation, you have difficulty breathing and the doctor places you on a respirator. Later your condition deteriorates and you are in a permanent coma. Can the doctor remove the respirator. In some states yes and others no. This dilemma was faced by the father of Dan Noel, the political columnist for the Hartford Courant (Figure 3-4).

Once a respirator or feeding tube is placed, whether it can be withdrawn or not depends on the circumstances and the state in which you live. Respirators are easier to withdraw from a legal and psychological point of view, because death occurs within minutes. A patient whose feeding tube is removed can languish for days before dying. In Appendix 2 is a summary of the current status of legal issues surrounding terminal care in each state. Some legal experts feel that the Supreme Court ruling regarding Nancy Cruzan renders unconstitutional any state restrictions on the withdrawal of feeding tubes and respirators in comatose patients.

After reading this, you probably have questions on how people prepare for death. Sixty-five percent of people who die do not even bother to make a will. Patients with health care proxies and living wills are few and far between. What generally happens is, the physician discusses the situation with the family and a decision is reached. Again, the main issue is trust.

SUMMARY

While a lot of publicity centers on comatose individuals being prolonged against their family's wishes, a consensus in the country is evolving that will make this a non-issue. The real fear is the slow inevitable deterioration that precedes dying. If you are coherent, there is no problem — you can assess your options and prognosis and decide for yourself if you want aggressive treatment. The problem is when a disease renders you mentally incompetent. A living will may make it

IS IT EUTHANASIA OR MURDER?

by Dan Noel

"You understand," said the doctor at the foot of Dad's bed, "that if you don't want us to ventilate your — force air into the lungs with a respirator — we won't. But once we start, we can't stop. Even if you're brain dead, we won't be allowed to stop." "I have to hear it from you. It doesn't matter what your family says — because it's your decision."

Mom and Dad long ago signed the Arizona version of living wills. They restated their intentions when he was rushed to the hospital a week ago Saturday night; the charts at the nursing station said clearly, "Do Not Resuscitate." The question of mechanically assisted breathing, however, had not been addressed.

I asked: "Might the occasion arise when a few hours' ventilation would help Dad through a crisis and not be needed again?" "Yes," the doctor said; "possible, although not likely." If the machine were used and didn't get Dad through the crisis, however, it could not be turned off.

Dad didn't hesitate. "Don't ventilate," he said.

He survived without a respirator. A mild heart attack damaged an already-weakened heart, but left him with all his faculties. Late last week, he was sent home with a new if uncertain lease on his 84-year-old life.

Dad probably wouldn't have faced that choice here; Connecticut's "death-with-dignity" protects doctors and hospitals that agree to discontinue ineffective treatment. Recent case law establishes the right of patients or delegated next-of-kin [health care proxy] to insist on pulling the plug — although one might have to change doctors or hospitals...

A friend asked, as I started west: Why had my mother called for the ambulance and emergency technicians? Dad's heart has been failing, a leaking mitral valve. They're reconciled to his going before her. Why not accept death?

The answer is in the 16 years they have enjoyed since Dad's first heart attack, and in the weeks or months or years they may yet enjoy after last week's relatively routine hospital measures.

One attempts the miracles modern-day medicine can perform. If there are to be no miracles, one accepts death-but not without trying.

Yet some- the prevailing view, apparently, in Arizona- would discourage trying;; withhold treatment for fear of having to withdraw it.

By what logic? Why should any human being be compelled to reject one dramatic therapy, lest it prove unsuccessful and he and his spouse of 60 years confined to living hell?

Dad's decision to refuse ventilation turned out to be moot. But what if he had accepted that option, and it proved fruitless?

Had a loving son then pulled the plug, it would have been called euthanasia by some, but murder in Arizona. Not, thank goodness, in Connecticut. Let's keep it that way.

The Hartford Courant. January 18, 1991. Reprinted with permission.

Figure 3-4

55

easier for your physician to respect your decisions and a health care proxy can further clarify your wishes. Make certain to provide your physician with copies of these documents and make provisions so your family knows where the originals can be found. If you make your wishes known without the use of these documents, your family can still refuse treatment but if the doctors or hospital disagree, get ready for costly, unpleasant and lengthy litigation. Anytime you walk into a court room even though the law may be on your side, to some extent, you have already lost. The emotional drain and legal expenses are devastating.

CHAPTER 4

DEGENERATIVE BRAIN DISEASES

The most tragic blow a person can suffer is loss of mental function. While physical disabilities are disheartening, the loss of mental function renders self-sufficient adults into helpless infants that require full-time assistance. Mental function or intellect involves many factors including memory, the ability to learn new skills, abstract reasoning, judgement, along with verbal and mathematical aptitude. Our consciousness, our ability to feel pain, our emotions – our essence – is because of our brain. When our brain dies, we die. When it slowly degenerates, so do we. Thus it comes as no surprise that patients are institutionalized more often for mental rather than physical problems.

Functions such as speech, walking and reasoning are localized in specific areas of the brain. For example after a stroke, a patient may suddenly lose his ability to speak but retain his writing skills. It is even

TESTS TO EXCLUDE REVERSIBLE DEMENTIAS

CAT scan of brain
EEG
MRI of the brain
Spinal tap
Blood tests to rule out metabolic disease (e.g. Glucose etc.)
EKG
Chest X-ray
Blood tests for anemia
Blood tests for nutritional deficiencies

Figure 4-1

COMMON REVERSIBLE CAUSES OF DEMENTIA

Medications - Virtually any medication can cause dementia
Depression and other psychiatric disorders
Alcohol
Poor sensory input - such as decreased hearing and sight
Lack of stimulation
Metabolic Disorders - e.g. Thyroid Disease, Diabetes
Tumors
Trauma
Infections
Poor nutrition
Syphilis

Figure 4-2

possible to lose one language skill and retain others. Immigrants who have had a stroke may lose their ability to speak English but still retain their native tongue. Degenerative brain diseases, on the other hand, generally result in a gradual but uniform loss of abilities. Many elderly view impaired mental function as a normal sign of aging. While memory and the ability to do complex math decline, reasoning and judgement are not impaired. Many people who live into their eighties and nineties remain alert and perceptive with sharp intellect. It is not a myth that wisdom comes with age. Even in ancient Egypt, where mental disease was treated by drilling a hole through the skull to release evil spirits — trephining — pharaohs retained their leadership positions into their nineties. While it is unlikely that trephining ever helped a mentally-impaired pharaoh, it resulted in his death so that a competent pharaoh could assume power.

*   *   *

When a precipitous decline in mental function occurs, a condition called dementia, it is imperative that a physician assess the patient and arrive at a diagnosis. Some causes of reversible dementia are listed in Figure 4-2 and the tests that may be performed to facilitate diagnosis are listed in Figure 4-1.

When the reversible dementias have been ruled out, the patient has an irreversible degenerative brain disease. While there are at least a dozen possibilities, in the United States, the following account for over 95% of the cases:

1. Alzheimer's Disease
2. Multi-Infarct Dementia
3. Parkinson's Disease
4. A combination of the above

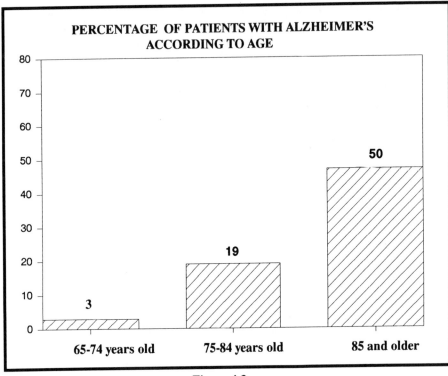

Figure 4-3

ALZHEIMER'S DISEASE

Alzheimer's, the fourth leading cause of death in the United States, is a relentlessly progressive brain degeneration that results in complete deterioration of mental function. It begins with memory loss, disorientation, personality changes and diminished communication skills. The patient then becomes unaware of his surroundings and is no longer able to recognize his family. Eventually, he becomes bedridden, incontinent, comatose and passes away.

The term Alzheimer's was once reserved for patients who developed dementia at an unusually young age, whereas the elderly demented were termed "senile" or given the diagnosis of "organic brain syndrome." This distinction stems from a political confrontation among physicians in the early 1900's. Doctors relish having their names attached to diseases just like politicians dream of having their names nobly engraved on a public edifices. Thus, Dr. Alzheimer successfully convinced the scientific community that early dementia was a separate entity from the well-known senility of old age. The present consensus, however, is that Alzheimer's is a single entity that usually presents in the elderly but occasionally is seen in people in their fifties and that it encompasses what previously was called senility. The number of neurofibrillary plaques in the brain seen in microscopic examination at autopsy, the hallmark of Alzheimer's, is correlated to the degree of dementia regardless of the Alzheimer's victim's age.

The devastation of Alzheimer's cannot be overstated. Two million people have Alzheimer's and it is estimated that almost 50% of people over 85 have early symptoms, although the vast majority in this age group are able to function (Figure 4-3).

A genetic basis for Alzheimer's has been elusive, but as diagnostic techniques improve, a greater familial predilection will be found. Already evidence is emerging linking Alzheimer's to specific chromosomes. Thus, never sign a long-term health-care insurance policy that excludes you on the basis of a family history of Alzheimer's. As the population ages, the majority of Alzheimer's victims may prove to have a positive family history.

Alzheimer's is often not diagnosed in its early stages because the initial symptoms are subtle and patients deny that they have a problem. It is suspected when there is a history of progressive dementia for which no other cause (as listed in Figure 4-2) can be found. The input of an internist, a neurologist and occasionally a psychiatrist is required. Unlike a brain tumor or thyroid disease, no specific test gives the diagnosis. Thus, physicians must rely on more subjective tests that evaluate mental function.

Mental function tests assess a variety of brain functions, but memory is preferred by physicians because it is independent of prior education and socioeconomic background. Memory is divided into three types: immediate, recent and remote. Alzheimer's patients initially retain their remote memory while losing immediate and recent memory. This is why early Alzheimer's victims have no difficulty recalling Babe Ruth's batting average in 1935, but can't remember where they put their shoes.

Recent memory lasts only for seconds and can store 5 to 9 datum. A typical test is the Digit Span test (Wechsler) in which sequences of numbers are given and the patient is asked to repeat them forwards and backwards. For example, the doctor says 3,5,9,2,7 and the patient is asked to repeat them. He then says 7,4,6,2,0 and the patient is asked to repeat them backwards. Most senior citizens can remember 4 digits forward and 3 digits backward. Those who cannot may have early Alzheimer's Disease.

Doctors also ascertain whether the patient is "oriented," — aware of who he is, where he is, and what time it is. Typical questions are:

> What season is it?
> What day is it?
> What is the date?
> What is your name?
> Where are you?
> Who is the president?

While these questions may seem simplistic, patients with Alzheimer's Disease have difficulty answering them. Tests that check for specific brain functions are a subspecialty in themselves and neurologists and psychiatrists are able to differentiate Alzheimer's Disease from the dementias that are due to other causes such as depressions and strokes.

Thus before a patient is given the diagnosis of Alzheimer's, a physician should first rule out the reversible causes of dementia and then do appropriate mental function tests. Even this approach is not 100% accurate in diagnosing Alzheimer's, but it is close.

Alzheimer's runs a predictable course. As can be seen from Figure 4-4, the average survival is four to five years from the time of diagnosis, although death can take as long as 10 years. Thus Alzheimer's, like metastatic cancer and AIDS, is a terminal disease. Being young, between 55 years old and 60 years old, does not improve the prognosis but aggressive medical treatment can prolong life. Affluent patients with Alzheimer's live longer because of better access to care. Thus, ironically, the poor afflicted with Alzheimer's may be more fortunate than the rich.

```
SURVIVAL RATE IN ALZHEIMER'S DISEASE

Years after diagnosis          % of patients still alive
         2                               85%
         4                               60%
         6                               40%
         8                               20%
```

Figure 4-4

*   *   *

Alzheimer's disease is divided into three phases that may overlap:

1. Confusional Phase. Patient can still function. The early Alzheimer's victim has minor annoyances because of memory loss. He does not remember where he left his keys, a friend's name escapes him, and he stops reading novels because he cannot follow the plot. His personality changes, usually for the worse. Driving in unfamiliar places becomes difficult and concern for his personal appearance diminishes. Confusion is sometimes worse at night, a phenomenon known to medical personnel as "sundowning."

As the disease progresses, the Alzheimer's victim finds it impossible to function in our complex society. Even the mentally healthy can be bewildered while programming a VCR, using an automatic-teller machine, dealing with a telephone-answering machine or fathoming income tax forms. The Alzheimer's victim is overwhelmed. Unsound financial decisions are made. A frugal elderly patient who survived the depression may donate a large portion of his life savings to a charity or religious denomination based on a single television advertisement. Bills go unpaid and Alzheimer's is often diagnosed by the worker who shuts off the victim's gas because of a delinquent account. Telephone-direct marketers love to prey on the elderly with early Alzheimer's and sell them useless health and life insurance policies or talk them into buying unnecessary items.

2. Dementia Phase. Patient can no longer function. At this point, the victim may become abusive, belligerent and physically violent as simple functions such as eating, dressing and bathing become impossible. Denial and lying are common. When he remembers to go to the bathroom, he forgets to clean himself. His elderly spouse must try to lift him from the commode to perform this task. As he is unfit to drive, the loss of this perceived right causes continued frustration. Inappropriate behavior such as sexual overtures to children and even public masturbation may occur. The victim becomes withdrawn and refuses to associate with old friends and family members.

3. Endstage. Patient requires full-time care. The patient is so disoriented that he must be watched constantly so that he does not wander and fall down a flight of stairs or trip. Caring for him is now a full-time job. There are no breaks and no vacations. The patient may even need to be heavily sedated or physically tied into a chair or bed unless his family can afford round-the-clock nursing care. He is now incontinent (unable to control his bowels and bladder), must be kept in diapers, and no longer recognizes anybody—even his own spouse. Eventually, he becomes totally bedridden and dies from either pneumonia, a bladder infection or infected bedsores.

*   *   *

There is no treatment for Alzheimer's. Often families with Alzheimer's victims become overly optimistic after hearing about a recent "breakthrough." Unfortunately, the medical community's understanding of Alzheimer's and the brain in general is still in the Dark Ages. A miracle cure is as likely as establishing a manned colony on Pluto. Many victims are mislead and buy low-Aluminum pans, bizarre and expensive lecithin diets and ineffective drugs with dangerous side effects. Depression in Alzheimer's can be ameliorated with medication but side effects such as increased disorientation and incontinence may occur. Even over-the-counter drugs or the intake of alcohol can cause a marked worsening of the dementia.

In summary, Alzheimer's is a relentless and hopeless disease that results in complete incapacitation of the victim and is eventually fatal.

There is no cure at this time. Alzheimer's victims generally fend for themselves for several years and then are relegated to a caregiver, either their spouse, daughter, or daughter-in-law. Those with no support structure quickly become wards of the state and are institutionalized. Given this information, some recommendations are in order.

Recommendations

If you are diagnosed as having Alzheimer's, you have the right to be treated with dignity and have your wishes respected. If you feel you do not want your life to be prolonged once your mental function has deteriorated, take the appropriate steps:

1. Face reality. Most people go through five distinct phases of denial, anger, bargaining, depression and acceptance when they receive news that their demise is inevitable. Try to get through the first four as quickly as possible. You cannot beat Alzheimer's and it is unlikely that the diagnosis is incorrect. I am not being insensitive. I'm just telling the truth.

2. Get your financial affairs in order. If you have significant assets, you must decide whether you want to retain your assets and pay for your own care or disperse them to your family. Remember that in most states, Medicaid restricts coverage for long-term care for 30 months after the last dispersal of assets. Please obtain good legal and financial advice quickly because as your disease progresses, complex decisions will become difficult. You may become paranoid and not trust anyone even though they are acting in your best interests. Designate someone to have durable power of attorney over your assets, especially if you are widowed or unmarried. Update your will and discuss your estate with your accountant or financial planner to minimize estate taxes.

3. If possible, obtain a long-term health care policy. The policy must specifically state that Alzheimer's, as a pre-existing condition, does not negate any of the benefits. Otherwise the insurance company will peruse your physician's records to see if Alzheimer's was diagnosed or even suspected. Then they will refuse to pay.

4. After checking the laws of your state (see Appendix 2), make your intentions clear. Sign a living will and assign a health care proxy. Make sure both of these documents are in your doctor's chart.

5. Find a nursing home that has a reputation for good care of Alzheimer's victims and place your name on its list.

6. You will have to decide for yourself whether you want aggressive treatment for other diseases such as cancer or heart disease. If you are only mildly confused and have a strong will to live, accept it. But remember, your Alzheimer's disease will not reach a plateau, it will continue to progress.

*   *   *

If you are the primary caregiver of an Alzheimer's victim, take the following steps:

1. Make sure you have durable power of attorney and are the health care proxy of the Alzheimer's victim.

2. Contact a local agency concerned with Alzheimer's. Meet with others who have been caregivers for Alzheimer's victims and hear firsthand the problems they have encountered. They will give you more insight and advice than any doctor, social worker, this book or any book for that matter. A good place to start is to look in your phone book for the local chapter of the Alzheimer's Disease and Related Disorders Associates, Inc. or else contact their national office at:

60 East Lake Street, Suite 600
Chicago, Il 60601
1-800-621-0379
1-800-572-6037 (Illinois only)

3. See what resources are in your local community. Many communities have support for the elderly such as transportation assistance, nutrition programs and adult day care. Try to obtain home-health care.

4. Do not become a martyr. Caring for an Alzheimer's victim cannot be explained; it must be experienced. Many books about Alzheimer's will tell you that caring is an act of love. For many, though, caring for an Alzheimer's victim becomes their worst nightmare fraught with feelings of anger and guilt and sometimes compounded with thoughts of violence towards the victim.

Initially, it is not too difficult, but as the dementia accelerates, it becomes a full-time and thankless job. The caregiver must realize that the loving person they remember no longer exists and nobody is to blame. Alzheimer's patients are often unappreciative and oblivious to their caregivers. You may even be struck, cursed at or spit upon. Do not wait until you feel angry and guilty. Find support groups and hire part-time care, even if you have to get a job to pay for it. It will help you cope with the situation. You must live your life too.

5. Institutionalize the Alzheimer's victim before you become overwhelmed. Even if you are financially secure and able to afford 24-hour care, Alzheimer's victims often become a danger to themselves and others. It can be emotionally traumatizing to see a loved one who is demented engaging in bizarre and inappropriate behavior. If the victim is incontinent, belligerent or wanders, you have already waited too long.

6. Do not place great faith in the medical profession's ability to help. For example, many caregivers are under the impression that after several tests, and a few pills, incontinence can be treated. Many books on Alzheimer's perpetuate this myth. Usually, these efforts are fruitless or offer only temporary relief.

7. Discuss with your doctor whether all the medications the Alzheimer's victim is taking are necessary. Putting medicine down the throat of an Alzheimer's victim and dealing with the concomitant side effects can be a trying experience. For example, hypertension is often treated with diuretics that cause the patient to urinate frequently. Other medications can cause diarrhea and vomiting. You have to clean this up. Blood thinners such as coumadin cause considerable demands on caregivers because the patient bruises easily and bleeds

profusely when shaved. Perhaps other medications can be used or else they can simply be discontinued.

8. Do not succumb to the fad of the day. Even if some miracle drug were discovered, by the time the FDA (Federal Drug Administration) approves it, your grandchildren will be retired. In Europe, where the regulations on the release of new drugs are much less cumbersome, no drugs have been found to be effective for Alzheimer's.

9. Do not force the Alzheimer's victim to eat. When the Alzheimer's victim turns his head at the sight of a spoon, he's sending a message. Leave him alone and allow nature to take its course. Alzheimer's is not painful and your loved one is not suffering. Placing a feeding tube for artificial nutrition is equally senseless.

10. When the Alzheimer's victim is permanently disoriented, consider refusing all care unless it is for comfort. Do not take him to the hospital and if he is in a nursing home, make sure they do not send him to the hospital. If he contracts pneumonia or a urinary tract infection, consider refusing antibiotics. If the nursing home refuses to honor your wishes, take him home. At this stage, home care is easier and the remaining days can be experienced with dignity. Hire visiting nurses to help you even if it may be expensive. It will preserve your sanity.

MULTI-INFARCT DEMENTIA

Multi-Infarct Dementia is the result of several strokes rather than a gradual global loss of mental function as is seen in Alzheimer's. However, there is considerable overlap with Alzheimer's and often both entities are combined in the same patient. Medical science does not have a comprehensive understanding of either disease and diagnostic confusion may result. It does not make any difference to the patient, though, because the average time of survival from the time of diagnosis is four to five years, similar to Alzheimer's. Multi-Infarct Dementia is associated with hypertension, but there is no evidence that treating the hypertension stops its progression. By and large, when a patient is given this diagnosis, follow the same guidelines for refusing treatment as with Alzheimer's.

PARKINSON'S DISEASE

In Parkinson's disease, a specific wiring system in the brain stops functioning. It often begins with a rhythmic trembling of the hands and arms and speech is impaired. The body then becomes rigid and the patient stoops over, shifting his center of gravity. This gives Parkinson's victims a characteristic gait in which they appear to be running to catch up with themselves. Unfortunately, the rigidity increases and these patients may become confined to a wheelchair or bedridden. Although this is not an inevitable consequence of Parkinson's, when this stage is reached, it is not reversible with medication or physical therapy. Full-time help or institutionalization is necessary. Endstage Parkinson's victims die from pneumonia, infected bedsores or urinary tract infections. The average life span from the time of diagnosis is 13 to 14 years.

When Dr. Parkinson described the disease in 1817, he stated that dementia was not a feature. Modern medicine now realizes that Parkinson's victims often have decreased mental function in 30% to 40% of cases but unlike Alzheimer's and Multi-Infarct Dementia, it is not inevitable. Parkinson's victims often have an emotionless face that belies their coherency.

With competent medical care from a neurologist, Parkinson's can be controlled but it still progresses in spite of treatment. Thus if you are diagnosed with Parkinson's, there is a reasonable chance that you will remain coherent and able to make your own decisions up to the very end. Nonetheless, you should designate someone with durable power of attorney and assign a health care proxy. Discuss your case and prognosis with your neurologist. Treatment is often effective for years but eventually, no medication helps. Your neurologist will be able to tell you when this happens with a high degree of accuracy. At this point, consider refusing all treatment that is not for comfort.

WHAT I WOULD DO IF I HAD A DEGENERATIVE
BRAIN DISEASE

In Parkinson's disease, I would accept treatment until my mental function had deteriorated or my neurologist felt it was futile. With Alzheimer's or Multi-Infarct Dementia, I would accept life-prolonging treatment in the early stages of the disease. I would leave directions in my living will and to my health care proxy that if I was afflicted with cancer, a heart attack, pneumonia or similar ailments, to refuse all treatment including antibiotics. I would not allow anyone with a feeding tube within a one-mile radius. I would not expect my family to care for me at home when I became hopelessly demented and would do whatever I could to see that my assets were used to make life easier for my family or donated to a favorite charity, rather than being spent on futile and prolonging care.

CHAPTER 5

COMAS AND STROKES

Unlike degenerative brain diseases, comas and strokes are sudden events that wreak havoc on previously orderly lives. Patients and their families are then plunged into a health care system that is dedicated to preserving life, but ill-equipped to deal with the emotional distress and physical decline that accompany these tragedies. Knowing when to refuse treatment is not always an easy decision, but some general guidelines are possible.

COMAS

A coma is a sleeplike unresponsive state brought on by disease, injury or poison (Figure 5-1). Considerable media attention and legal discussions center upon the unfortunates in prolonged comas, or in the current vernacular — persistent vegetative states. Debates and court decisions make national headlines; however, persistent vegetative states are rare.

In a given year about 50,000 patients become comatose and half of them die within 48 hours. Forty percent have a complete or partial recovery, 7 percent die later and only 3 percent remain in a persistent vegetative state (Figure 5-2). There are less than 15,000 patients in persistent vegetative states in the United States and while this is tragic for the victims and their families, in a country of a quarter-of-a-billion people, it is not a problem many people are forced to confront. The chance of being in a persistent vegetative state is less than the chance

COMMON CAUSES OF COMA

1. Mass lesions in the brain (tumors, blood, abcesses)
2. Strokes
3. Infections (e.g. meningitis)
4. Trauma
5. Poisons (e.g. drug overdoses, chemical imbalances)
6. Brain degenerations (e.g. Alzheimer's)

Figure 5-1

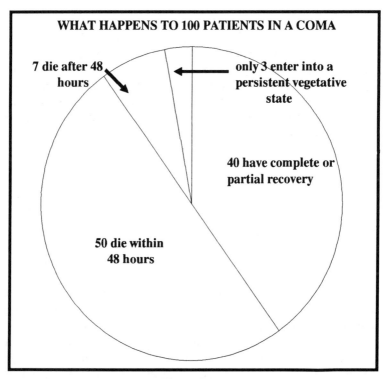

WHAT HAPPENS TO 100 PATIENTS IN A COMA

7 die after 48 hours

only 3 enter into a persistent vegetative state

40 have complete or partial recovery

50 die within 48 hours

Figure 5-2

of being dealt a straight flush. Nevertheless, comas themselves are common and a familiarity with them can greatly reduce anxiety.

The brain is organized so that the higher centers that control our intelligence, personality and emotions — our consciousness — are located in the upper portion, the cerebral cortex. The lower portion of the brain — the brainstem — regulates our vital organs: the heart, lungs and kidneys. Evolution has furnished humans with a system that preserves the life-sustaining portions of the brain, the brainstem, even at the expense of the cerebral cortex. For example, if the brain is deprived of oxygen for a brief period, the cerebral cortex may die but the brainstem can survive. The patient loses consciousness, but still has respiratory function. That is, the brain is still giving commands to the lungs to keep the body alive.

Thus, comas fall into one of three categories:

1. Total brain death
2. Brainstem function only
3. Brainstem and partial cerebral cortex function

What classification a patient falls into cannot always be ascertained immediately. It may take several weeks or even months to formulate a diagnosis.

Total Brain Death

Total brain death can be diagnosed with complete accuracy by use of an electroencephalogram (EEG), a machine that measures the electrical activity in the brain. This instrument led to the Harvard definition (Figure 5-3), in which, after certain stipulations, two EEG's that show no brain activity indicate brain death. Patients in this category can only be kept "alive" with a feeding tube, a respirator and round-the-clock nursing care.

There is no difference between total brain death and death. The brain-dead patient has no consciousness or ability to feel pain. Thus a brain-dead patient connected to a respirator, an intravenous line and a feeding tube is in some ways similar to a corpse. For the patient's family, though, it is a horrible ordeal emotionally and possibly finan-

```
┌─────────────────────────────────────────────────────────┐
│                                                         │
│       HARVARD MEDICAL SCHOOL DIAGNOSIS OF BRAIN         │
│            DEATH IN COMATOSE PATIENTS                    │
│                                                         │
│   1. Totally unresponsive                               │
│   2. No movements or breathing                          │
│   3. No reflexes                                        │
│   4. No brain activity on EEG on two readings 24 hours apart │
│   5. Source of coma is not hypothermia or drug overdose │
│                                                         │
│                                                         │
└─────────────────────────────────────────────────────────┘
```

Figure 5-3

cially. A health care proxy or family member could consent to have the respirator disconnected so that "death" will follow its natural course. The laws of most states make this relatively simple.

Brainstem Function Only

When the brainstem is functioning, a respirator is not always necessary. Consciousness is irreversibly gone and from a practical point of view, there is no difference from total brain death; however, the patient may be able to breath on his own. Nancy Cruzan and Karen Ann Quinlan were classical examples of this category. Unlike total brain death, the EEG shows brain activity, but a feeding tube, hydration and round-the-clock nursing care must be maintained to keep the patient "alive." After a neurologist has ascertained there is no reasonable hope for recovery, tube feedings and hydration could be terminated. Again, in most states this is not difficult, but unlike discontinuing a respirator, "death" can take several days.

Brainstem and Partial Cerebral Cortex Functioning

Comatose patients with both brainstem and cerebral cortex functioning present difficult ethical dilemmas as there is a vast variation in their ultimate outcome. The recuperative powers of a damaged brain can be phenomenal, especially in the young; however, neurologists are not always able to accurately predict the final outcome early in the coma. A patient's family may become frustrated and angry with their neurologist when a loved one has a recent-onset coma because the neurologist has little inkling as to the final outcome. Virtually all coma victims who survive for two to four weeks show some signs of awakening. This sometimes gives families false hopes.

Neurologists have been trying for decades to determine what signs are accurate in predicting who will recover from a coma. Many protocols have been established and all of them incorporate the following: age, reason for the coma, extent of brain damage and the period of time in the coma.

1. Age. For reasons that are not clearly understood, the young brain has greater recoverability. Victims of head trauma who are less than 20 years old have a higher incidence of rehabilitation than older victims. Children have a remarkable capacity to recuperate from massive brain injury.

2. Reason for the coma. Patients with comas secondary to low body temperature—hypothermia—or from a drug overdose have a good prognosis. Notice how the absence of these two conditions is necessary for the Harvard definition of brain death (Figure 5-3). A primitive reflex, the diving reflex, may allow a youngster to remain submerged under water for up to 45 minutes without irreversible brain damage. When the face hits the cold water first, the body shunts virtually all blood to the brain and the cold water permits the body to use energy more efficiently. Thus, if a patient is in a coma from a drug overdose or hypothermia, the coma should be reversed when there are no longer any drugs in the blood, or when the temperature has returned to normal. If it does not, there is a higher chance that the coma is irreversible. On the other hand, comas secondary to strokes, brain degeneration and oxygen deprivation have a poorer prognosis.

3. Extent of the brain damage. Patients who are completely paralyzed and whose pupils do not react to light have a poor prognosis.

4. Time in a coma. This is one of the best prognosticators. In general, the longer one is in a coma, the less the chance for recovery. After three months of a coma, there is little chance of recovery and after a year, it is practically non-existent.

*   *   *

Coma victims who wake up often have permanent brain damage. Remember from Figure 5-2 that the vast majority of those who survive the first 48 hours do wake up. Many have personality changes that make them combative, argumentative and paranoid.

Holding a steady job is often impossible, even if they are capable of menial labor. Some regain consciousness but are bedridden. They must be turned to prevent bedsores, given tube feedings, have their diapers changed and have mucous suctioned from their throat to prevent pneumonia. Even the smartest neurologist cannot predict which patients will end up in this state.

If you are uncertain about terminating care in a comatose loved one, you have time. Permit your doctors to place a feeding tube while waiting for recovery. In most states, it can be removed if your doctor and you agree at a later time that your loved one's condition is irreversible (see Appendix 2).

What I Would Do If a Family Member Were in a Coma

If our neurologist was able to diagnosis total brain death or only brainstem function, I would have the hospital discontinue the feeding tube and respirator. This determination may take time and it is possible that our neurologist may never see the specific EEG findings or physical signs to accurately diagnosis brain death. In this case, I would obtain the second opinion of another neurologist but not expect either one to give me a specific timetable for when to stop tube feedings and other treatments.

I would be willing to wait a month in the case of an older person but up to six months in the case of someone younger, my 30-year-old brother for instance. Financial factors would have to be considered also. The care of a coma victim can easily eclipse $20,000 a month. If our insurance or the government were covering the care, I would be patient. However, I would not deplete the life savings of my family on the remote possibility that a loved one may recover from a coma.

STROKES

Sad but true, people in the midst of leading full lives can be devastated by a stroke. Although high blood pressure and cigarette smoking are risk factors, no one is safe. Often there is no warning and a healthy, happy person can be pummeled by this juggernaut, forever rearranging his life and that of his loved ones.

A stroke occurs when a portion of the brain is deprived of oxygen resulting in a physical or mental deficit that persists for greater than 24 hours. This differs from a temporary deficit that resolves completely within 24 hours — a "transient ischemic attack" or TIA.

Strokes or "shocks" have a wide variation. Some are so small that they result in barely perceptible personality changes while others result in total paralysis or death. A stroke can cause a variety of deficits but below are the more common ones:

- one-sided paralysis of either the arm or leg or both
- inability to speak
- inability to speak clearly
- inability to understand speech
- inability to read
- inability to write
- loss of peripheral vision
- personality changes
- loss of short-term and/or long-term memory
- urinary and fecal incontinence
- a combination of the above

The clinical presentation of most strokes is so striking that they are easily diagnosed by examining the patient, although a CAT scan or MRI is done for confirmation. In spite of extensive research, medicine

77

has made little progress in aiding stroke victims. For most patients, rehabilitation is the only option.

Care of stroke victims has three phases: the acute phase, the maintenance phase and the convalescent phase.

The acute phase. During the acute phase, the main goal is to keep the patient alive. Strokes have a mortality rate of 20% to 30% and this has not improved in the past 30 years. Strokes are the third-leading cause of death in the United States.

An attempt is also made to keep the stroke from spreading. Blood thinners such as heparin and coumadin are given, although many doctors feel they are of dubious efficacy. Paralyzed limbs are positioned and moved daily to prevent permanent contractures.

The convalescent phase. When the patient is medically stabilized, the convalescent phase begins and the focus is on rehabilitation. With luck, the stroke may begin to resolve, although no medical treatment will aid this. For example, a patient who is paralyzed on one side and unable to speak may notice improvement in arm and leg coordination. His previously garbled speech starts to become coherent. Sadly, though, this is not always the case. Rehabilitation involves actively attacking the deficits with physical and speech therapy. It may be highly successful in motivated patients, even if there is no resolution of the stroke. Those paralyzed on one side usually relearn how to walk, although fine hand movements are permanently lost. Speech therapy is not as successful, but often does wonders for the patient's psychological well-being.

The maintenance phase. Improvement, either from the stroke itself or due to physical therapy, is rare after six months and after this point, patients should not be given false hopes. Further attempts at rehabilitation are usually futile and the patient is now in the maintenance phase and permanent deficits must be addressed. Patients who do poorly are those with the inability to walk, urinary and fecal incontinence and poor motivation.

*　　　*　　　*

Thus, strokes are catastrophic events in which after six months, there is virtually no hope of functional improvement. Patients who cannot speak, never will. Patients bound to wheelchairs will remain there. Often, the media will dramatize the plight of a highly-motivated individual who courageously overcomes the conservative medical establishment and persists in overcoming a horrible stroke. While this may be theoretically possible, patients given false hopes often end up feeling deluded, bitter and hostile towards their doctors and other caregivers.

As in Alzheimer's, the patient's family is quickly overwhelmed in caring for a stroke victim. The workload is not only physically awesome but psychologically draining. Stroke victims often have personality changes and become self-centered and demanding, leaving the caregiver to feel inadequate, unappreciated and exhausted.

Again, the key to deciding whether or not to refuse treatment is self-awareness and will to live. Stroke victims often have speech impediments and apathetic facial expressions that belie a sharp intellect. One of my patients is unable to speak but still plays a mean game of bridge. Other stroke victims vacillate between lucidity and confusion. Unlike Alzheimer's patients, a stroke victim will not continue to deteriorate rather he will reach a plateau, usually by six months. This is the time to assess whether it is possible to care for the patient at home or whether institutionalization is necessary. With present medical technology, it is possible to keep a stroke victim alive for decades.

Patients who are self-aware can decide for themselves whether to pursue treatment based on their will to live. Life-threatening conditions such as pneumonia and urinary tract infections are common in these patients. For example, assume you are wheelchair-bound, unable to speak and require assistance to eat and use the bathroom. You may still enjoy life and have the financial resources to have yourself taken care of without rearranging the lives of your loved ones. You may still enjoy reading and watching television. On the other hand, you may feel that your earthly sojourn is over and prefer to see doctors only when watching Quincy reruns.

If you decide you do not desire any treatment, assert yourself. No doctor can give you antibiotics or place you in the hospital unless you consent. You have the right to refuse treatment. Your family should respect your decision and not try to have psychiatrists declare you incompetent. It's a free country. Some doctor may diagnose you as being depressed and recommend some potion to cure your depression. Remember, you have reason to be depressed. You are bound to a wheelchair and cannot communicate efficiently. You are dependent on others for your sustenance. No doctor can change this. If you lose your appetite, you can elect not to have artificial nutrition via feeding tubes or hyperalimentation.

Patients who have lost their self-awareness are a difficult dilemma. Since they are not terminal, they can remain confused but healthy for years. Depending upon the degree of impairment, some can be cared for at home while others need institutionalization. The decision to place a stroke victim in a nursing home has no formula, but the main issue is incontinence. Incontinent patients quickly overwhelm any family that is not fortunate enough to afford full-time nursing care. Some books compare caring for this type of individual to caring for an infant. This is complete nonsense. Caring for an infant is much easier. When an infant soils himself, you simply pick him up and change him. Unless you are Hulk Hogan, this is difficult to do with an adult. Many adults become hostile at the indignity of being wiped and changed after soiling themselves. The interests of the patient and family may be better served if the patient is placed in a nursing home or in an extended adult day care facility.

What about refusing treatment for this type of individual? Even if the patient has a living will, in most states it is technically not valid because he does not have a terminal disease. What about the rights of a health care proxy? Can a health care proxy refuse life-preserving care in a confused non-terminal patient? If you ask five legal scholars this question you will probably get ten different answers. I do not pretend to know how to solve this difficult dilemma, but families facing this situation should be aware of one thing: if you take such a patient to a doctor, do not expect the doctor to respect your wishes and not treat him. The doctor could not only be exposed to a malpractice charge, but also manslaughter. If you do not want him treated, do not take him to a doctor or to a hospital emergency room.

What I Would Do (And Hope My Wife Would Do) If I Had a Stroke

I would accept aggressive medical treatment and rehabilitation for six months. At this point, I would reconcile myself to the fact that my condition is not going to improve. As long as I was enjoying life and not making life miserable for my family, I would accept aggressive treatment for short-term life-threatening conditions such as pneumonia, appendicitis or a urinary tract infection. I would accept any treatment that improves my quality of life such as cataract surgery. On the other hand, if I developed terminal cancer or endstage heart disease, I would only accept treatment that controls pain. If I felt I was too dependent on my family to the point where the lives of others had to center around me, I would refuse all treatment including antibiotics. If the stroke left me demented, I would hope my wife or health care proxy would refuse all treatment except for comfort. I would not want to be within a five-mile radius of any doctor or hospital.

CHAPTER 6

CORONARY ARTERY DISEASE

Tremendous strides have been made in the treatment of heart disease but it still accounts for 38% of deaths in the United States – the leading killer. While there are a multitude of heart problems, this chapter will confine itself to the largest with no close second – coronary artery disease. Its major manifestations are angina (chest pain) and heart attacks.

The underlying problem in coronary artery disease is the deposition of fats and calcium – atherosclerosis – in the coronary arteries, the blood vessels that supply oxygen to the heart (Figure 6-1). These depositions can also block blood vessels in any organ such as the brain (strokes), kidneys, or eyes. Thus, coronary artery disease is a subclass of a much broader abnormality, atherosclerosis, that is poorly understood and ineffectively treated. While eating healthy foods and exercising regularly may be helpful, atherosclerosis has a strong genetic component. Every doctor has patients in her practice who are 90 years old, never heard of cholesterol or low-impact aerobics and go into fits of uncontrollable laughter at the suggestion they stop eating red meat.

Coronary artery disease does not occur suddenly or even over a matter of years, rather it is a disease that percolates for decades. The best way to explain this is by an example. Please refer to Figure 6-2 which shows the progression of coronary artery disease in a typical

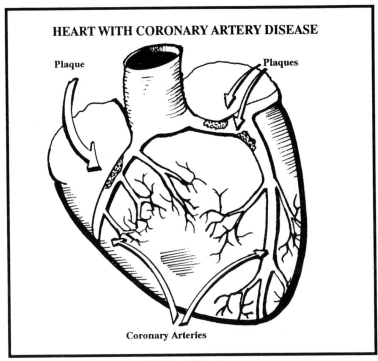

HEART WITH CORONARY ARTERY DISEASE

Plaque

Plaques

Coronary Arteries

Figure 6-1

patient, Mr. Wilson. At age 40, small depositions – plaques – begin to deposit in Mr. Wilson's coronary arteries. The most accurate method of diagnosing his coronary artery disease is by performing a cardiac catheterization, a procedure in which dye is injected into the coronary arteries and X-rays are taken to visualize the plaques. Since there is no treatment at this stage of the disease and cardiac catheterizations can have side effects, Mr. Wilson's doctor sees no sense in obtaining one. Ten years later, Mr. Wilson has a stress test during a routine physical. In a stress test, the patient is asked to walk on a treadmill that is similar to that seen in any health club except that it costs ten times more. His doctor, by examining Mr. Wilson's cardiogram during the stress test, sees evidence of coronary artery disease. He asks Mr. Wilson if he has chest pain or shortness of breath and Mr. Wilson replies he does not.

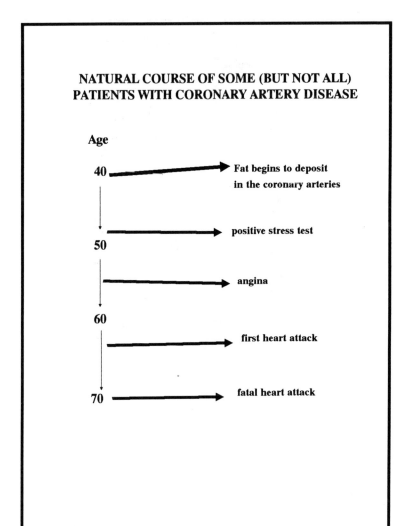

NATURAL COURSE OF SOME (BUT NOT ALL)
PATIENTS WITH CORONARY ARTERY DISEASE

Age

40 — Fat begins to deposit in the coronary arteries

50 — positive stress test

60 — angina

— first heart attack

70 — fatal heart attack

Figure 6-2

Seven years later, Mr. Wilson has chest pain while mowing his lawn. His internist prescribes nitroglycerin tablets to place under his tongue when the pain occurs. As this relieves Mr. Wilson's symptom, his internist does not perform further tests. Even though his coronary arteries now have significant blockage, Mr. Wilson's internist feels that subjecting him to the small but significant risk of a heart catheterization will not change his treatment.

At age 65, Mr. Wilson has his first heart attack. He stays in the hospital for ten days and has no complications. Further testing reveals that no further treatment is warranted. At age 70, Mr. Wilson has a second heart attack that results in his immediate death.

This sequence is not engraved in stone. Many patients with coronary artery disease never experience chest pain and their first manifestation of heart disease is a heart attack. Diabetics may not have chest pain even when having a heart attack! Everyone has heard of the supposedly-healthy patient who has just received a clean bill of health from his internist only to succumb to a heart attack a week later.

Some patients with coronary artery disease are warned by angina — chest pain — caused by a temporary lack of oxygen to the heart. Doctors diagnose angina by observing its abatement to nitroglycerin, the same compound used to make dynamite. Unfortunately, other types of chest pain, such as that caused by spasm of the esophagus, also respond to nitroglycerin. Thus the gold standard in diagnosing coronary artery disease is cardiac catheterization, although it is not 100% accurate.

If you are given the diagnosis of angina, do not assume you have one foot in the grave. Coronary artery disease manifested by angina has a low annual mortality rate. While it is obviously better not to have coronary artery disease, if you are a 50-year-old man, you have a 50% chance of living to be 63 years old. A 70-year-old man has a 50% chance of living to be 78.* Women have an even better prognosis.

The goal of treatment is to either eliminate the angina or diminish its frequency so that the patient is not a cardiac cripple. The first line of attack is medication, but if disabling angina persists, angioplasty or bypass surgery is recommended. In angioplasty, a balloon is used to

* The 70-year-old man has a shorter life span than the 50-year-old man because he has a higher chance of dying from other diseases.

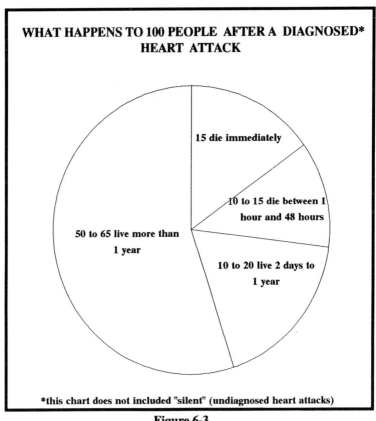

WHAT HAPPENS TO 100 PEOPLE AFTER A DIAGNOSED* HEART ATTACK

15 die immediately

10 to 15 die between 1 hour and 48 hours

50 to 65 live more than 1 year

10 to 20 live 2 days to 1 year

*this chart does not included "silent" (undiagnosed heart attacks)

Figure 6-3

dilate the coronary arteries. In bypass surgery, the diseased coronary arteries are replaced with veins from another part of the body. The problem is that neither dilating the diseased coronary arteries nor a sophisticated plumbing operation corrects the underlying problem, atherosclerosis. Even with new coronary arteries, the plaques still redeposit. For this reason, bypass surgery and angioplasty do not prolong life in many cases.

The media and politicians are constantly whining about the cost of so-called unnecessary bypass surgery. Other countries, such as Canada and England, restrict access to bypass surgery. What is not said is that this wonderful procedure has greatly enhanced the quality of life of millions. Patients who could not climb a flight of stairs without chest pain and shortness of breath can resume playing tennis. In good hands, bypass surgery has a 1 percent to 2 percent mortality rate and a 80% to 90% 5-year survival rate – not bad at all. The same policy makers who complain about its cost are the first people to be wheeled into the operating room when something is wrong with their ticker.

A more ominous manifestation of coronary artery disease is an occlusion of a coronary artery that kills a portion of the heart muscle – a heart attack. This results in immediate death in 15% of the cases and of those who survive, another 10% to 15% die within 48 hours of the attack. Thus only 70% to 75% of people with a heart attack survive 48 hours (Figure 6-3).

The survival of those hospitalized has risen dramatically in the past two decades, thanks to improved drugs, refined surgical techniques and coronary care units. Prior to these advances, 30% of patients hospitalized for a heart attack died; today less than 10% die.

The damage from a heart attack can be limited by quickly administering a drug that dissolves the occlusion in the affected coronary artery. The patient is then placed in intensive care for the treatment of lethal abnormal heart rhythms should they occur. If the chest pain persists, a cardiac catheterization searching for potentially-lethal blockages of the coronary arteries should be done. If one or more are found, the patient often has immediate bypass surgery or angioplasty.

If you survive your first heart attack do not start lining up your pallbearers. A patient alive one year after an uncomplicated heart attack has a fairly good prognosis – only a 5 percent annual mortality rate. This means a 50-year-old patient who has just had an uncomplicated heart attack has 50% of living to be 61 years old. A 70-year-old patient has 50% chance of living to be 77 years old. However, notice the key word here – UNCOMPLICATED.

There are several complications of heart attacks – valve damage, strokes, aneurysms of the heart wall, heart failure and abnormal heart rhythms. Blood thinners may prevent a stroke and unless your cardiologist has wax in his ears, he will hear a valve abnormality with his stethoscope and have it fixed surgically. The two common ones, though, abnormal heart rhythms and congestive heart failure, are the big killers.

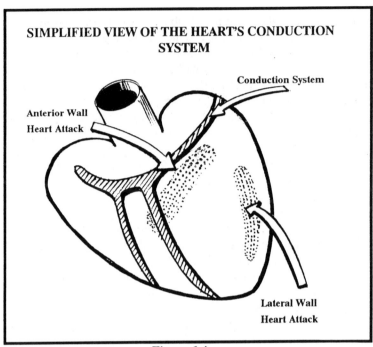

SIMPLIFIED VIEW OF THE HEART'S CONDUCTION SYSTEM

Conduction System

Anterior Wall
Heart Attack

Lateral Wall
Heart Attack

Figure 6-4

Abnormal heart rhythms or arrhythmias occur when the wiring (conduction) system that choreographs the heart's four chambers into beating efficiently malfunctions. A graphic display of the heart's electrical activity is called an electrocardiogram (EKG) and cardiologists dedicate their entire careers to the study of the subtle blips that differentiate benign and malignant arrhythmias and how best to treat them. Please look at Figure 6-4 which shows a simplified view of the heart's conduction system. Remember, in a heart attack part of the heart muscle dies and this includes the cells that comprise the heart's conduction system, causing arrhythmias. Arrhythmias are treated with medications, pacemakers and in some cases surgery. The most significant development in cardiology in the past decade has been the creation of implantable defibrillators with miniature computers that detect malignant arrhythmias and administer an electrical shock to return the heart to a normal rhythm.

Some types of heart attacks rarely cause arrhythmias. Again please look at Figure 6-4. When the highlighted anatomical area labeled the lateral wall is damaged by a heart attack, the chance for a malignant arrhythmia is small because the major branches of the conduction system are spared. In England, lateral wall heart attacks are not even admitted to a hospital because statistically speaking, hospitalization does not alter their course. On the other hand, an anterior wall heart attack (again see Figure 6-4) has a much greater chance of disrupting the conduction system. How do you know if your arrhythmia is a lethal one? Well, if you are alive one year after your heart attack, it was either a benign or treatable arrhythmia. It's really that simple.

The other major complication of a heart attack is congestive heart failure. This occurs when so much heart muscle has been damaged that the heart cannot muster a strong contraction. Thus, oxygen-giving blood is circulated poorly, resulting in decreased energy. Patients with congestive heart failure are classified according to the amount of activity they can perform prior to experiencing symptoms:

- Mild - patient has symptoms with moderate physical activity such as during a brisk walk or climbing stairs
- Moderate - walking can cause symptoms
- Severe - Patient has symptoms even at rest

These patients also have episodes where fluid backs up in the lungs, resulting in shortness of breath. Doctors diagnose this problem by hearing the fluid in the lungs with a stethoscope or seeing the fluid on a chest X-ray.

The severity of the heart failure often correlates to what cardiologists refer to as the "ejection fraction." Please look at Figure 6-5. The normal heart ejects 55% to 70% of its blood into the circulatory system with each contraction and this percentage can be determined by a cardiac catheterization or a heart scan. After a heart attack, this percentage often decreases. A heart attack that damages a small amount of heart muscle may not result in a significant change in the ejection fraction, but a massive heart attack can cause a precipitous lowering of the ejection fraction. Ejection fractions lower than 20% are barely compatible with life.

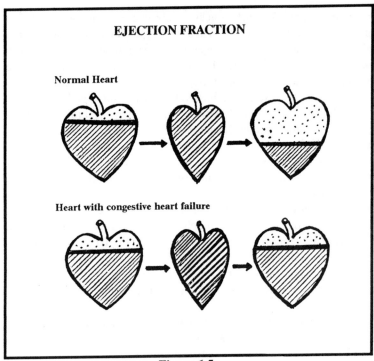

EJECTION FRACTION

Normal Heart

Heart with congestive heart failure

Figure 6-5

Why am I making a big deal about the ejection fraction? Because it correlates highly with a heart failure patient's prognosis. As can be seen from Figure 6-6, the lower the ejection fraction, the worse the prognosis. Please look at the dismal prognosis of a heart failure patient with a 20% ejection fraction — a 45% annual death rate. This patient has a poor chance of surviving three years. While this chapter has emphasized coronary artery disease as a long-term entity spanning decades, patients with severe congestive heart failure have a terminal disease like patients with metastatic cancer and AIDS. These patients do not need sophisticated tests and brainy cardiologists with thick glasses to tell this to them. They know it because they are miserable. They can not carry a bag of groceries without becoming short of breath and walking up stairs becomes a herculean task.

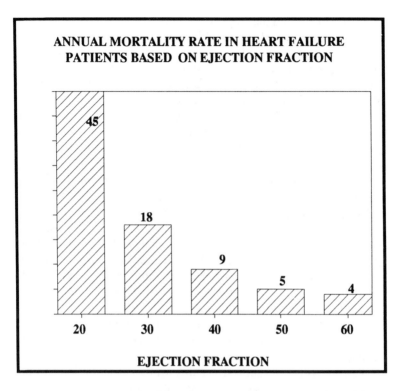

ANNUAL MORTALITY RATE IN HEART FAILURE PATIENTS BASED ON EJECTION FRACTION

Figure 6-6

The medical treatment of congestive heart failure centers on diuretics to decrease the amount of fluid in the body and medications such as digoxin and dobutamine which increase the strength of the heart's contractions. While it does not prolong life, treatment enhances the quality of life and patients do not look like fluid-filled orbs when they pass away as they did before these drugs were developed. Some patients are even staying at home while receiving intravenous dobutamine. There are some data to indicate that a class of medications called vasodilators, which reduce the work the heart performs, are helpful in endstage heart failure, although at best they may give several months of additional life.

More aggressive treatments are also available. Some cardiologists recommend dialysis for severe heart failure. While the details of this treatment are beyond the scope of this book, suffice it to say that it has not been proven to prolong life, although it can reduce the number of episodes a patient will suffer shortness of breath due to excess lung fluid. Balloon pumps are sometimes temporarily inserted in the largest blood vessel, the aorta, to help the heart beat more efficiently. Again, this may help a patient temporarily recover from an episode of shortness of breath, but it does not reverse the problem—an inefficient heart. Heart transplants are curative but donor hearts are rarely available and are reserved for younger patients with no other health problems. Experimental surgical techniques that reinforce the heart with muscle taken from other parts of the body are being developed and my hat is off to the brave patients who consent to them. Attempts to develop artificial hearts have thus far been unsuccessful.

A patient with severe congestive heart failure has increased incidences of episodes where he becomes short of breath. Unless he refuses treatment, he may spend the final months of his life going in and out of the hospital until the inevitable occurs. With each hospitalization, he is given higher doses of diuretics, digoxin and dobutamine. If these medications are ineffective, the patient must be intubated and placed on a respirator. If he cannot be weaned, he spends his final days with a tube down his throat in constant agony until he dies.

Patients with endstage heart failure are often under the impression that they will die a hideous death from suffocation. This is rarely the case. Almost 50% of those with endstage heart failure die from an arrhythmia, a painless and practically instantaneous death. The remainder enter a semi-stupor in which breathing is labored but there is not a choking sensation.

Thus, when you have endstage heart failure, you need to decide when to stay away from the doctor and the hospital, otherwise you may be prolonged and uncomfortable. You have the advantage of having good mental function so you can rationally decide when you want to refuse treatment.

SUMMARY

Coronary artery disease can be a long-term chronic disease with a good prognosis or a rapidly fatal one. Those with angina but no history of a heart attack have an excellent prognosis regardless of whether or not they need bypass surgery to control their symptoms. Patients who are alive one year after a heart attack have an excellent prognosis unless they have congestive heart failure. In this case, the prognosis can be crudely predicted according to the ejection fraction. Patients who can barely walk accompanied by low ejection fraction have severe heart failure — a terminal disease. As mental function is not affected, they may opt for themselves whether they desire treatment.

WHAT I WOULD RECOMMEND IF MY FATHER HAD CORONARY HEART DISEASE

As long as he did not have terminal congestive heart failure, I would have him accept the treatment recommended by his cardiologist. If he was unfortunate enough to be severely incapacitated by congestive heart failure and had an ejection fraction between 20% and 25%, I would not recommend he be hospitalized unless he was in pain. Although there may be some benefit in using dialysis, balloon pumps and surgical muscle transpositions, I would not recommend them as they would be painful and/or inconvenient and at best give only several additional weeks of life. I also would not recommend he be intubated and placed on a respirator.

CHAPTER 7

CHRONIC OBSTRUCTIVE LUNG DISEASE (COPD)

In the first week of my internship, I was introduced to a patient with severe emphysema. The chief resident told me that I would be seeing this gentleman frequently for the rest of the year. He was right. By the end of my internship, I had known him and dozens of other emphysema patients on a first-name basis. They came into the emergency room — terror in their eyes — breathing rapidly as they tried to get air into their diseased lungs. I intubated them, blasted them with a variety of potions and within a week or two, they returned to their homes. A month later, they were back with the same look of terror. The cycle could not last forever and most of them died.

Emphysema is a horrible disease and like patients with congestive heart failure, they have a predictable prognosis. Aggressive treatment gives them several months of life, perhaps more, but not much more. Emphysema is part of a spectrum of lung diseases called chronic obstructive pulmonary disease (COPD) that also includes chronic bronchitis. Much ado is made about the difference between these two entities, emphysema being characterized by a gaunt patient breathing heavily, while in bronchitis, the patient is constantly coughing and producing sputum. In actuality, these two entities overlap and for all

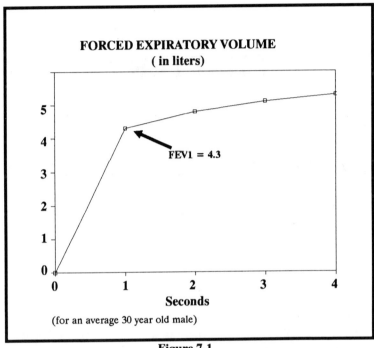

Figure 7-1

practical purposes, COPD is air hunger that is the result of lung damage from cigarette smoking.

If you are diagnosed as having COPD, there are three things you must do. This first of these is to stop smoking. Secondly, you have to stop smoking. Third and most important, you must stop smoking. Early in the course of COPD, the cessation of smoking may stop the progression of the disease and actually permit the improvement of lung function. Unfortunately, if the COPD is advanced, the cessation of smoking will not prevent the COPD from getting worse, although it may do so at a slower rate.

Your doctor will monitor your lung function with pulmonary function tests. You are asked to blow rapidly into a tube that is connected to a machine that measures the volume of air expired over a period of time, a spirometer. This results in a graph similar to the one depicted in Figure 7-1. Please bear with me while I explain this.

SURVIVAL IN A COPD PATIENT

FEV1	Average Life Span	2-year survival	5-year survival
1.25 liters	7 years	90%	80%
0.75-1.25 liters	about 6 years	82%	55%
0.50-0.75 liters	2-3 years	65%	33%
0.50 liter	1 year	35%	10%

Figure 7-2

The horizontal line (or X-axis for you math fans) represents the amount of time in seconds. The vertical line (the Y-axis) is the volume of air expired. In this patient, 4.3 liters of air was expired in one second. This is called the forced expiratory volume or FEV1. A simplified analogy would be to see how large you can blow up a balloon in one second. Normally, an average-sized 30-year-old male can expire 4.3 liters, about 4 quarts. This diminishes with age but an unaffected older person still has an FEV1 of 3.2 liters or about 3 quarts.*

If you have COPD, your airways are obstructed and you expire less air. Your FEV1 is decreased, depending on how many cigarettes you smoke a day, how many years you've been smoking and how your lungs respond to the cigarettes. Even before the spirometer was invented, physicians knew that a COPD patient had the inability to exhale large amounts of air rapidly and tested him be having him attempt to blow out a match held one foot away from his mouth.

Why am I explaining the FEV1? Because if you have COPD, it is a fairly accurate predictor of your symptoms and prognosis. Please look at Figure 7-2. By knowing your FEV1, you have some indication of your expected life span. If your FEV1 is above 0.75 liter your expected life span is reasonably good. Once the FEV1 is under 0.75 liter, though, you are approaching the end of your life. More important

---

* Purists may note that I am interchanging the volume of gas with the volume of a liquid. Under normal conditions, both occupy the same amount of space.

SIGNS THAT COPD IS IN THE TERMINAL PHASE

1. Chair bound
2. Rapid weight loss
3. FEV1 of 0.75 liter or less
4. Need to be intubated

Figure 7-3

is how you feel. If you have no energy, no appetite and are losing weight, you have reached the terminal phase of COPD (Figure 7-3).

Perhaps an example will make this a little clearer. Please take a look at Figure 7-4 which compares Mr. Smith, a non-smoker, and Mr. Jones, a smoker. At age 20, both of these men have good lung function and an FEV1 of 4.5 liters. However, because Mr. Jones begins smoking at this time, his FEV1 and his lung function decrease at a much more rapid rate so that by age 35, his FEV1 is 3.2 liters, equivalent to Mr. Smith's at age 80! But look at the chart again. Most patients do not have symptoms of lung disease such as increased sputum production and shortness of breath until their FEV1 is less than 2 liters. So when Mr. Jones' doctor tells him to stop smoking because he already has lung damage, Mr. Jones politely nods, grabs his golf clubs, plays 18 holes, and continues with his two-pack-a-day habit. Notice on the chart that if Mr. Jones had stopped smoking by age 40, his FEV1 would still decrease but never to the point where he developed symptoms of lung disease. This is why the cessation of smoking is so important.

When Mr. Jones is 50 years old, he has a problem. He gives up walking the golf course and rents a cart. When he hooks a ball into the woods, he does not bother to chase it. Mr. Jones now concludes that his doctor was not a complete bozo after all and quits smoking. Look what happens to his FEV1 in Figure 7-4! It keeps on decreasing, but at a much slower rate. If he is lucky, it may decrease at a slow rate, but he now has COPD and will have to live with it the rest of his life. The only cure is a new set of lungs. On the other hand, if Mr. Jones never stops smoking, in 5 to 10 years, his FEV1 will be around 0.75 liter and he will be miserable. He will have a new friend, his oxygen tank. Golf

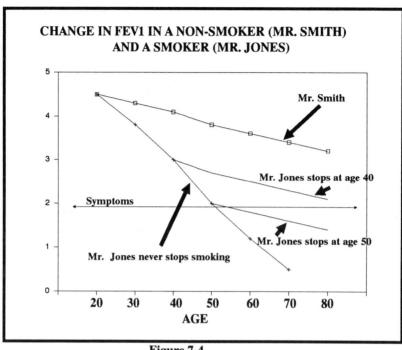

**CHANGE IN FEV1 IN A NON-SMOKER (MR. SMITH)
AND A SMOKER (MR. JONES)**

Mr. Smith

Mr. Jones stops at age 40

Symptoms

Mr. Jones stops at age 50

Mr. Jones never stops smoking

AGE

Figure 7-4

will be a thing of the past since he can't even muster up the energy to get out of his cart, let alone swing his driver. As his COPD worsens, he will become housebound and may end up so short of breath that he cannot even walk.

Patients who stop smoking have a worse prognosis than those who do not. Why is this? It's because when they finally decide to stop, their FEV1 is around 0.75 liter and they cannot pick up their grandchildren without becoming short of breath. Even if their lung function diminishes every year like that of a non-smoker, they are still going to do poorly. In other words, those whose COPD has made them so miserable that they finally stop smoking, are too sick to recover. Those with just mild symptoms of COPD are not motivated enough to discontinue smoking.

Treatment of COPD revolves around medications to improve respiratory function, antibiotics to stamp out frequent infections and

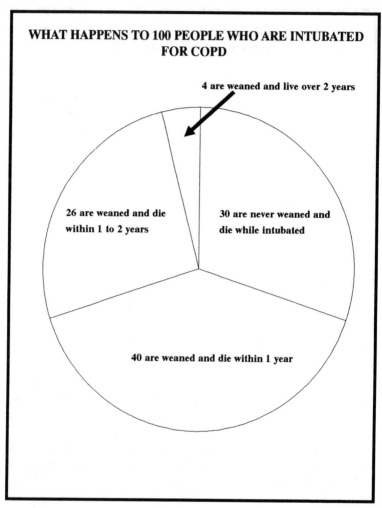

Figure 7-5

supplemental oxygen administration. While these regimens can abate symptoms they do not reverse the declining lung function. The main fear of COPD patients is that they will die a hideous death from suffocation. This is rarely the case. COPD patients slip quietly into a coma and have a comfortable peaceful death if nature is allowed to take its course. A major question that all patients with COPD must address is whether they want to be intubated.

The need to be intubated in itself is an indication that a patient's COPD is entering the terminal phase (Figure 7-3). Please look at Figure 7-5 which shows what happens to 100 patients who require intubation for COPD. Thirty percent of them cannot be weaned from the respirator and of those who survive, most are dead within one year.

But look at this chart carefully. Twenty-six patients survive over one year and four survive over two years. Is there any way to predict who will do well with intubation and who will not? No, but by and large, patients with a low FEV1, recent weight loss and no energy have a poor prognosis and often do not survive even when intubated. In other words, those who survive do so because their underlying disease is not as severe.

If you insist on a full-court press when your COPD enters the terminal phase, you can have a miserable death. What happens is, you go into the emergency room and the emergency room doctors do their job. They see that you are having difficulty breathing and put you on a respirator. Now comes the problem. Your doctors must wean you, but if your lungs are endstage, it is not possible. You just stay on the respirator, sometimes for weeks, until a heart attack or infection ends your life. Again, look at Figure 7-5. This happens to 30% of patients intubated for COPD. If you become comatose and live in a state where it is possible to remove the respirator, you are lucky. However, if you are still mentally alert, no doctor will be willing to turn off the respirator and watch you die. The sight of a terrified elderly patient attached to a respirator is one of the most disconcerting in all of medicine.

Thus, when you reach the terminal state of COPD, consider avoiding emergency rooms and hospitals. Your home or a hospice is the place to be. Home care for COPD patients has greatly improved. Portable oxygen tanks make it possible for ambulation and even visits outside the home. There are even light-weight liquid oxygen systems that can be carried on your back. They are expensive and you are going to have to pull teeth from Medicare and your insurance company to pay for them. Studies have shown that home-oxygen therapy can improve quality of life and even increase life span. Most of the medications and therapy can be given at home. It is even possible to have a portable respirator in your house that can attach to a hole in your windpipe when you are having breathing difficulties. Many hospitals and communities have wonderful pulmonary rehabilitation programs that help patients and their families cope with this disease. Information on the best care available in your community may be obtained from:

Emphysema Anonymous, Inc.
P.O. Box 3224
Seminole, Fl 34642
813-391-9977

American Lung Association
1740 Broadway
New York, NY
212-315-8700

SUMMARY

COPD is an ugly disease that has a predictable prognosis. Patients go through a declining level of activity, from independence to being housebound to being unable to get out of a chair. Patients with a low FEV1, rapid weight loss, and no energy are terminal. Patients must decide whether they desire intubation. Terminal-COPD patients often have a more comfortable and dignified death if they stay at home or in a hospice and avoid emergency rooms and hospitals.

WHAT I WOULD DO IF I HAD COPD

I would accept aggressive treatment including intubation as long I was able to walk and had enough energy to leave my house. Once I became chair-ridden, emaciated and my FEV1 was below 0.75 liter, I would refuse to go to the hospital and have myself taken care of at home with the medication and oxygen that my doctor recommended. I would not permit myself to be intubated. As my life span would be limited to another 1 to 3 years at best, I would not accept aggressive treatment if I were to develop other medical conditions. If my dependence became too demanding on my family, I would enter a hospice.

102

CHAPTER 8

CANCER

The war on cancer has been in the public eye for the past generation and has resulted in phenomenal successes. Some types of
leukemias, Hodgkin's disease and testicular cancer can be cured even
in advanced stages. Unfortunately, the common adult cancers such as
lung, colon, stomach, and breast are still deadly unless they can be
surgically removed before they have spread. To this day, the major
methods to combat cancer are prevention and early detection.

More people than ever are dying of cancer. Presently, cancer
causes 30% of the deaths in the United States and those in their thirties
and forties have a 50% chance of dying of cancer. Thus, dealing with
cancer is a problem many will face. The reason for this phenomenon
is an ongoing debate in the medical community, with some doctors
blaming increased environmental carcinogens while others postulate
that improved treatment of infections, lung disease and cardiac disorders has increased cancer deaths by the process of elimination.

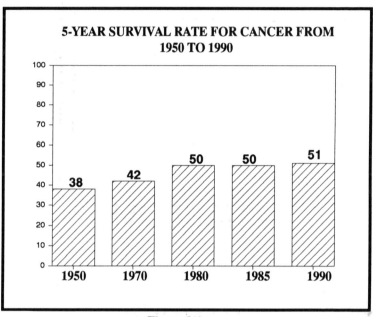

Figure 8-1

Whether significant progress against cancer has been made is another raging debate in the medical community. While there is unanimity that most cancers cannot be cured, there is a large divergence of opinion as to whether treatment prolongs life and if so, whether the rigors and side effects of that treatment are worth the additional months. Please consult Figure 8-1. Notice that from 1950 to 1990, the 5-year survival rate of cancer victims increased from 38% to 51%, a change of 13%. Some physicians believe this demonstrates improved treatment modalities. Others point out that better diagnostic equipment and greater access of the general public to medical care has resulted in cancers being diagnosed earlier.

There is also a huge variation in the mortality rates of different types of cancer. Please review Figure 8-2. While patients diagnosed with pancreatic cancer die quickly, those with endometrial (uterine) cancer are usually alive 10 years after diagnosis. Thus, cancer for many is a chronic disease.

5-YEAR SURVIVAL (%)

Site of Cancer	1950	1975	1980	1990
Esophagus	5	5	5	8
Stomach	12	15	16	17
Colon	41	50	52	56
Rectum	40	48	50	53
Liver	4	4	3	4
Pancreas	3	3	3	3
Throat (larynx)	60	65	66	67
Lung	6	12	13	13
Skin melanoma	56	79	81	81
Breast	60	74	74	76
Cervix	59	68	67	65
Uterus	72	88	84	82
Ovary	30	36	38	39
Prostate	43	66	71	73
Testis	55	78	88	92
Bladder	53	72	75	78
Kidney	35	52	52	52
Brain	16	22	24	25
Thyroid	80	92	92	94
Leukemia	10	33	35	35

Figure 8-2

As Mark Twain noted, there are lies, damn lies and statistics. While some may view these data as evidence that we are winning the war against cancer, in actuality, little progress has been made in the past 40 years. Unless the tumor can be completely removed surgically, before it has metastasized (spread to other organs or lymph nodes), treatment often results in giving the patient several more months of life that may be painful and debilitating.

For example, refer to Figure 8-2 with reference to lung cancer. In 1950, 6 percent of patients survived five years. In 1990, the 5-year survival increased to 13%. It could be argued that today's treatment is more effective. But look at these numbers with common sense. How often did people go to the doctor in 1950 and how many of them had chest X-rays? Today, a doctor will order a chest X-ray for a hangnail. Thus, lung cancer may be fortuitously diagnosed at an earlier state when it may be cured by removing it. Colon cancer, a frequent killer, had a 40% 5-year-survival rate in 1950 and by 1990, the 5-year-survival rate increased to 53%. In 1950, colon cancer was diagnosed at a later stage. Usually the patient had a large tumor that was obstructing his colon so that he could not have a bowel movement. The surgeon opened him up, found the tumor and informed the patient to get his affairs in order. Now with modern medicine, doctors who are the least bit concerned about colon cancer will pass a tube up the colon — colonoscopy — and search for tumors. Many patients with no symptoms have colonoscopy done as part of a routine physical. Obviously, some colon cancers will be found at an earlier stage. This is the main reason the 5-year-survival rate has improved, not because of better treatment.

Just to play devil's advocate, assume that the improved survival is because of better treatment. Even with this scenario, only a fortunate few benefit. Return to the example of lung cancer. If 5 people out of 100 survived for 5 years in 1950 and 13 people out of 100 survived for 5 years in 1990, then only 8 out of 100 had improved survival. Thus, the odds of this being you is 1 out of 12, worse than the chance of filling an inside straight.

While many American doctors will not agree with my analysis, doctors in other industrialized countries do not treat cancer aggressively. In Japan and Russia, doctors do not even inform patients they have cancer because they believe it causes undue anxiety. Emperor

Hirohito was never told by his doctors that he had cancer. Obviously, this approach is unacceptable in our consumeristic society; however, patients do have the right to know that their prognosis is poor and may want to consider forgoing the rigors of radiation therapy and chemotherapy and allow nature to take its course. Very rarely, if ever, is a patient with a common type of cancer cured with chemotherapy or radiation therapy.

*　　*　　*

Cancer occurs when a cell goes awry and replicates at an astounding rate. This can happen in any body tissue and by the time most cancers are symptomatic, the tumor is comprised of billions of cells. Chemotherapy and radiation therapy are primitive, brute-force attempts to kill these rapidly reproducing cells. This is rarely possible and only infrequent types of cancers such as Hodgkin's Disease, testicular cancer and some leukemias have been cured by these modalities. These treatments also attack normal cells that replicate rapidly such as those that manufacture hair and intestinal cells responsible for food absorbtion. This is why the common side effects are hair loss, diarrhea and nausea.

Nonetheless, most cancers will be cured some day. Research is being directed at finding characteristics that are unique to cancer cells. Antibodies specific only for cancer cells will then be manufactured in a laboratory and injected into the patient. While this technology is in its infancy, future doctors will someday view chemotherapy and radiation therapy the way we now view blood-letting.

When cancer is suspected, a doctor will biopsy the suspicious area. For example, in suspected breast cancer, a biopsy of the tumor is performed. If microscopic examination of the tissue by a pathologist (a doctor who specializes in examining body tissues and doing autopsies) shows cancer, the physician then determines how extensive the cancer is by a process called "staging." This is a sophisticated system involving multiple diagnostic tests in which a team of physicians looks at the size of the tumor, whether it has spread (metastasized), what organs it has spread to, and the degree of malignancy (Figure 8-3). Also there are subclasses of tumors depending upon the cell type. For example, with skin cancer, a tumor that comes from the protective part

```
┌─────────────────────────────────────────────────────────┐
│                                                           │
│     COMMON TESTS TO SEE IF CANCER HAS SPREAD              │
│                                                           │
│        CAT scan or MRI of head                            │
│        Bone marrow biopsy                                 │
│        CAT scan of abdomen                                │
│        Chest X-ray                                        │
│        Liver-Spleen Scan                                  │
│        Biopsy of Lymph Nodes                              │
│        Staging Laparotomy                                 │
│                                                           │
│                                                           │
└─────────────────────────────────────────────────────────┘
```

Figure 8-3

of the skin called the epidermis has a much better prognosis than one that comes from the cells that are responsible for skin pigment, the melanocytes. A negative staging work-up does not assure the patient that the cancer has not spread because these tests are incapable of detecting small metastases. Thus, a doctor who surgically removes a tumor may tell the patient he "got everything," but rarely will he be in a position to promise a cure.

Doctors can estimate the prognosis and longevity of a patient based on the stage. While there are large variations depending on the kind of cancer, some general concepts apply:

1. Complete surgical removal of a tumor without evidence of recurrence or metastases after several years is considered a cure.

2. Metastatic or recurrent cancers generally prove to be fatal. The average time of death is 15 months and some doctors feel that treatment with traditional medical therapy does not increase life span.

Cancer can cause death suddenly by precipitating a massive infection or a hemorrhage, but this typically, is not the case. Usually, the patient simply enters a terminal phase characterized by rapid weight loss and weakness—terminal cancer syndrome (Figure 8-4). The

POOR PROGNOSTIC SIGNS IN CANCER (TERMINAL CANCER SYNDROME)

poor appetite
rapid weight loss
shortness of breath
inability to perform activities of daily living

Figure 8-4

patient's prognosis is grave whether rich or poor, black or white, male or female, treated or untreated. Patients with terminal cancer syndrome are short of breath, have a poor appetite and are unable to perform the activities of daily living such as bathing and eating. Most are dead within four months and the number who survive eight months is less than 1 percent.

Often these poor patients are subject to artificial feeding by gastric tubes and hyperalimentation. They are placed in intensive care units, hooked to numerous monitors and tormented with ritualistic laboratory tests and X-rays. A good doctor will recognize when a patient has terminal cancer syndrome and redirect her treatment towards keeping the patient comfortable so that the patient's final days are dignified, pain-free and do not bankrupt the family. Patients with terminal cancer rarely belong in the hospital and are much more comfortable living out their remaining days at home or in a hospice.

If you have terminal cancer syndrome, you and your family should not insist that "everything be done." Do not expect your doctor to perform miracles and do not give her the impression you will sue her or report her to the State Board of Health. You need to establish a dialogue with your physician in order to receive maximum benefits from her professional expertise.

Patients with incurable cancer often require pain control. Not only is it possible to give analgesics and narcotics to suppress pain, but the nerves that transmit the pain impulses can be deadened. Sophisticated techniques have been developed whereby injections of anesthetics are administered into the nerves under the guidence of CAT scans and ultrasounds. Catheters can be placed near the spinal cord and anesthetics can be injected when pain becomes intolerable, the same way obstetricians deaden the nerves when performing a Caesarian section. These wonderful modalities can make a patient's final days pain free, but are probably not used often enough.

*   *   *

While this chapter cannot discuss all the cancers, it will discuss the more common ones. The key point to remember is to discuss your situation with your doctor. There are no absolutes in cancer treatment. Every patient has different goals and expectations. Only you, the patient, can decide the goals of your treatment and at what point to discontinue treatment. Some patients may be willing to tolerate any amount of treatment if there is a possibility that they will get several more months of life, so—for example—they can spend their last Holiday season with their families. Other patients may be simply want to let nature take its course.

While there are many exceptions, a good general guideline is that if you have metastatic or recurrent cancer, treatment at best will give several more months of life. Most oncologists, especially those in private practice, will level with you. They know your prognosis, whether treatment will help your symptoms, and when you have entered the terminal phase. Chemotherapy and radiation therapy, while rarely curative, can sometimes prolong life, alleviate pain and make your final days easier and more comfortable.

LUNG CANCER

Lung cancer can only be described as an epidemic paling all other cancers in frequency. The prognosis for lung cancer is directly related to the stage with one exception, a tumor called oat cell (small cell) carcinoma. This tumor responds well to chemotherapy regardless of the stage, but only a minority of patients are still alive one year after the diagnosis. The average survival of a patient diagnosed with the more common variety of lung cancer (squamous cell) is six to nine months and only 20% are alive after one year. With aggressive treatment, survival may be increased by several months, although the data substantiating this are dubious at best.

The staging system of lung cancer is complicated and at the risk of outraging the oncologists, I have simplified it (Figure 8-5). Those who survive Stage 1 are the fortunate ones in which the tumor can be completely removed. Lung cancer rarely causes symptoms when small

---

SIMPLIFIED STAGING SYSTEM OF LUNG CANCER

Stage 1 - Tumor is only in the lung
Stage 2 - Tumor has spread to nearby lymph nodes
Stage 3 - Tumor has metastasized to another organ
(e.g. liver, brain, etc.)

APPROXIMATE PROGNOSIS ACCORDING TO STAGE

	% alive after 2 years	Average survival
Stage 1 (lung only)	45 %	25 months
Stage 2 (lymph nodes too)	25 %	7 months
Stage 3 (other organs too)	10 %	5 months

Figure 8-5

and by the time the patient presents to his doctor complaining of a cough or blood in his sputum, the tumor is the size of a golf ball and has spread to his lymph nodes and other organs. The lucky ones are those who have a chest X-ray for an unrelated reason and a small tumor is noted and removed before it has metastasized. After surgery, there is no evidence to indicate that chemotherapy or radiation therapy improves longevity.

Again, I am going to upset the oncologists, but by and large Stage 2 lung cancer is treated with radiation therapy and Stage 3 is treated with chemotherapy. The protocols established are incomprehensible and vary depending on the institution and doctor. Neither of these treatments can prolong life for more than several months, but they may enhance comfort. The tumors may shrink after treatment but are not completely eradicated. The average survival of a patient treated with radiation therapy and/or chemotherapy is five to seven months.

What I Would Recommend If My Father Had Lung Cancer (Squamous Cell Variety)

1. In Stage 1 lung cancer, I would recommend surgery if his surgeon believed complete removal of the tumor — a cure — was possible. If his surgeon thought the tumor was inoperable, I would have him refuse chemotherapy and radiation therapy unless he was uncomfortable. In some instances, radiation implants can relieve pain.

If he had surgery but the tumor recurred in his lungs, the attempt at a cure had failed and further surgery would be futile. If the tumor recurred in his lymph nodes or at a distant site such as the liver or brain, his initial staging was incorrect, but the tests were not precise enough to detect the spread. This is a frequent occurrence. I would recommend he have no further treatment except to make him comfortable.

2. If he had Stage 2 (local spread) lung cancer, I would have him accept one session of radiation treatment. I would have him refuse further treatment unless he did exceptionally well with the first treatment. There is a syndrome seen in lung cancer patients in which the neck and face become swollen because the tumor blocks blood

drainage from these areas. It often responds dramatically to radiation therapy or chemotherapy.

3. With Stage 3 (metastatic to distant organs) lung cancer, I would have him refuse any treatment that was not for symptom relief. For example, if the tumor spread to his brain and caused severe headaches and deterioration of mental function, I would have him take a course of radiation treatment. Although it would not cure him, it may shrink the tumor, relieve the symptoms, and make his final months more dignified.

COLON CANCER

Colon cancer, the biggest cancer killer of non-smoking males, often progresses slowly and those with metastatic disease can survive for years. Some researchers believe that aggressive treatment prolongs life while others are of the opinion that while treatment can enhance patient comfort, it does not improve longevity. The colon is the last five feet of the intestine and includes the rectum. Thus, for the purpose of this discussion, rectal cancer is included as colon cancer. Like lung cancer, colon cancer is often diagnosed after it has spread. Common symptoms are weight loss, poor appetite, diarrhea, constipation and blood in the bowel movements. Numerous staging systems have been devised, but little improvement has been made on the one described by Dr. Dukes in 1932 (Figure 8-6).

When colon cancer is suspected, the tumor is demarcated with a barium enema, a procedure in which dye is placed in the intestines and X-rays are taken. A tube is passed up the colon and a biopsy is performed. If cancer is found, a further work-up including CAT scans and liver-spleen scans are done to see if the cancer has metastasized. If no metastases are found, an attempt is made to surgically remove the tumor. During the procedure, the colon often must be attached to the wall of the abdomen, a colostomy. Thus, patients must wear a bag under their shirt to collect the oozing fecal material. The lymph nodes are also biopsied. Notice from Figure 8-6 that a positive lymph node biopsy (i.e. cancer is in the lymph node) places the patient in the Dukes C stage and diminishes the prognosis.

If the tumor is metastatic to the liver, lung or brain (Dukes D), treatment may prolong life by several months but death is inevitable. This does not mean you should refuse treatment. Colon cancer can sometimes block the colon, making bowel movements impossible. This is extremely painful and can lead to bowel perforation and a quick death. Thus treatment should be accepted if your doctor considers bowel obstruction to be a probable event. Colon cancer may invade the nerves of the lower back, causing extreme pain. Spinal anesthesia often works wonders.

```
DUKES STAGING SYSTEM OF COLON CANCER
AND SURVIVAL WITH CURRENT TREATMENT

         Description                    5-Year Survival

Dukes A  Tumor is in inside wall of colon           82%
Dukes B  Tumor extends to outside wall of colon     73%
Dukes C  Tumor has spread to local lymph nodes      45%
Dukes D  Tumor has metastasized to other organs     25%
```

Figure 8-6

What I Would Do If I Had Colon Cancer

If the staging procedure showed that the cancer was metastatic to distant organs (Dukes D), I would refuse all treatment, including surgery, except for comfort. For example, if I had colon cancer that had metastasized to my liver or lungs, I would refuse all treatment except for pain control.

If my surgeon felt a surgical cure was possible, I would accept it only after a lymph node biopsy was negative, even if I had to undergo two surgical procedures. I would not want to deal with the inconvenience and risks of surgery along with the annoyance of a colostomy unless a cure was possible.

With Dukes A or B (the tumor is confined only to the colon), I would accept an attempt at a surgical cure and consider postoperative chemotherapy or radiation therapy if my oncologist thought that it might give me several extra months of comfortable life. If the tumor recurred, I would not accept further surgery unless my physician felt a bowel obstruction or another debilitating complication was likely.

BREAST CANCER

Breast cancer is a leading killer of women and one out of nine women will cope with this disease. While progress has been made in the treatment and palliation of patients with this entity, non-surgical treatment rarely results in a significant increase in life span. Referring to Figure 8-1 again, you can see that in 1950, 60% of patients diagnosed as having breast cancer were alive five years later and today that percentage has increased to 76%. This is not a substantial improvement, especially in light of early detection methods.

Unlike other cancers, breast cancer has wide variations in aggressiveness. Some patients have an indolent form of breast cancer that allows them to survive over 10 years, even with metastatic disease. Others have a virulent variety that steals their lives in a matter of months. Thus, staging is not as relevant to prognosis as in other cancers. Breast cancer also differs from other cancers in that it is often visible without doing X-rays and biopsies. The natural history of the disease was established in nineteenth-century England before doctors tried radiation therapy, chemotherapy or even surgery. Doctors from that era discovered that some breast cancer patients survived over 15 years. Today, the patient surviving into her second decade after treatment is held up by the medical profession and the media as a triumph of modern science. However, it is entirely possible that this patient simply has a less aggressive type of breast cancer and would have done just as well without treatment.

Early breast cancer appears as a mass or is noticed on a screening mammogram. Patients with metastatic breast cancer may complain of bone pain or headaches, depending on where the tumor has spread. Once suspected, a biopsy is performed and if it is positive, a metastatic work-up is done including palpation of the lymph nodes in the axilla (armpit). If the tumor has spread, breast removal is rarely productive and radiation, hormonal and/or chemotherapy is given for palliation. No cure has been definitely recognized. If the tumor is not metastatic, an attempt is made to cure the disease. The techniques

**10-YEAR SURVIVAL IN BREAST CANCER AFTER RADI-
CAL MASTECTOMY WITHOUT CHEMOTHERAPY OR
RADIATION THERAPY**

Nodes negative	80%
Nodes positive	40%
1-3 nodes positive	55%
4 or more nodes positive	25%

Figure 8-7

used depend upon the surgeon's philosophy and experience, along with
the patient's wishes. Some doctors favor mastectomy in which the
entire breast is removed while others prefer a "lumpectomy" followed
by radiation therapy, in which the tumor is removed but the breast is
preserved. For tumors that have spread to the muscles of the chest, a
radical mastectomy, where parts of the chest wall muscles are removed,
is recommended. In all these procedures, the lymph nodes in the axilla
are usually biopsied to see if the cancer has spread.

If you have breast cancer, you will constantly be faced with choices
of whether to accept or refuse treatment and when you accept it, what
type and how much. If the cancer is confined to the lymph nodes and
breast tissue, your prognosis without treatment is listed in Figure 8-7.
Patients who have no cancer in their lymph nodes do extremely well.
Even those with positive lymph nodes have significant survival. Some
data indicate that patients with only one to three positive lymph nodes
have increased survival with chemotherapy. On the other hand, postoperative radiation therapy has been shown to decrease local recurrence but it does not change survival. Also, radiation treatment to the
axillary lymph nodes may cause the patient's arm to irreversibly swell.

There is a subset of breast cancer that is called "receptor-positive" that adds another dimension to treatment. In these patients, a
receptor on the tumor causes rapid growth when exposed to estrogen,
a hormone prevalent in women. Treatment is either to block estrogen
with medications or surgically remove the ovaries, which secrete
estrogen. In receptor-positive breast cancer, hormonal treatment

reduces symptoms because the tumor(s) shrink. The cancer still exists, though, and there is no proof that survival is increased.

Metastatic breast cancer at the time of diagnosis is a terminal disease, but some patients live for years without treatment. Common sites of metastasis are the bones and brain, where their effects can be horrible. Breast cancer in the bones may respond to hormonal treatment. Breast cancer that spreads to the spinal cord can result in paralysis and loss of continence. Radiation therapy can be a godsend as can spinal anesthesia. Brain metastases can cause mental deterioration and intractable headaches.

Recurrent breast cancer is incurable whether it is metastatic or recurs in the breast or chest wall after an attempted surgical cure. The average survival time after recurrence is two years, but can range from weeks to several years. The time between the first diagnosis of breast cancer to the finding of a recurrence is called the disease-free interval. A short disease-free interval has a dire prognosis. For example, a patient has a mastectomy and is supposedly cured. One year later, a new tumor is found in the area where she had the mastectomy. Her prognosis is grave because the tumor recurred so quickly. On the other hand, a similar patient may have a metastasis to her hip bone six years later. Obviously, she has a less virulent type of breast cancer and her stay of execution will be longer. There is no evidence that any type of treatment changes the prognosis in either of these patients.

What I Would Recommend If My Wife Had Breast Cancer

If the tumor was metastatic and had the appropriate tissue receptors, I would recommend she take hormone treatments. I would have her refuse chemotherapy and radiation therapy unless she was in pain, such as in the case of bone or brain metastases.

If she did not have metastatic disease, I would recommend the surgical approach that had the greatest chance for cure, making cosmesis a secondary issue. If only one to three lymph nodes were positive, I would have her accept one course of chemotherapy but no radiation therapy unless her oncologist strongly disagreed. If the breast cancer recurred, I would have her accept hormonal therapy if she had receptor-positive disease, but have her consider refusing other treatment unless it was to make her comfortable.

PROSTATE CANCER

Prostate cancer is the male equivalent to breast cancer because it is common, may respond to hormonal treatment, and often has a slow progression allowing some patients with metastatic disease to survive for years. The most common symptoms are difficulty with urination or pain in the back and pelvic areas. With improved screening procedures, many asymptomatic patients are being diagnosed with prostate cancer, giving rise to difficult medical dilemmas.

The prostate gland is located at the base of the bladder and aids in sperm production. Doctors assess the prostate gland by doing a rectal exam. When a patient's symptoms or routine rectal examination makes prostate cancer a diagnostic possibility, an ultrasound followed by a needle biopsy of the gland is performed. If the biopsy is positive, the cancer is staged.

The staging of prostate cancer is complex and at the risk of incurring the wrath of my urological colleagues, I am going to simplify it (Figure 8-8). In Stage 1, the cancer has not spread and the tumor is subclassified according to size, location and degree of malignancy. In Stage 2, where the tumor has spread to the lymph nodes, and Stage 3, where the tumor has spread to other organs, the substage is not relevant because the tumor is already metastatic.

Prostate cancer metastasizes to the bones, liver, lungs and brain although any site is possible. Thus, the staging work-up includes a CAT scan of the head, a liver-spleen scan, a chest X-ray and a bone scan. If any of these tests are positive, the patient has Stage 3 prostate cancer. If they are negative, most urologists will recommend a biopsy of the lymph nodes near the prostate. If any of these nodes have cancer, the patient is placed in Stage 2. If these tests are all negative, the patient has Stage 1 prostate cancer.

There is an ongoing debate among urologists and oncologists on whether to initiate treatment of Stage 1 prostate cancer and if so, what modality is most effective. The problem is that with the increasing number of screening rectal examinations, followed by accurate ultrasounds and needle biopsies of suspected tumors, a large number of asymtomatic cases of Stage 1 prostate cancer are being discovered. You may say, "What problem? The cancer is diagnosed early. Why not remove it before it spreads?"

SIMPLIFIED STAGING SYSTEM FOR PROSTATE CANCER

Stage 1 Tumor is localized to the prostate gland or surrounding tissues.

Substage A1 - Tumor cannot be felt with rectal exam and has a low grade of malignancy when biopsied.

Substage A2 - Tumor cannot be felt with rectal exam but has a high grade of malignancy when biopsied

Substage B - Tumor is felt only in the prostate gland itself.

Substage C - Tumor can be felt beyond the prostate gland

Stage 2 Tumor has spread to the lymph nodes
Stage 3 Tumor has spread to other organs

Figure 8-8

The answer is that treatment of prostate cancer has never been proven to increase life span and can have serious side effects. A patient's prognosis is based on the stage and degree of malignancy of the tumor, not the treatment rendered. Please refer to Figures 8-9 and 8-10. Thirty percent of those over 80 years old and older have asymptomatic prostate cancer! Also notice that the 15-year-survival rate of Stage 1 prostate cancer is over 75%. Obviously, the vast majority of patients 80 years old and older will die from another disease before their prostate cancer affects them. Thus, aggressive treatment is rarely recommended in this age group.

In younger patients, the issue of the treatment of Stage 1 prostate cancer is not so clear-cut. Tumors that are Subclass A1 are not treated unless they cause symptoms by impinging on the urinary tract. In this case, a procedure called a transurethral resection (TURP to friends)

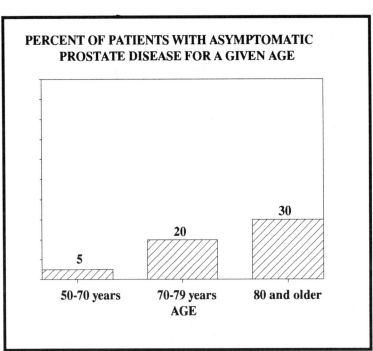

**PERCENT OF PATIENTS WITH ASYMPTOMATIC
PROSTATE DISEASE FOR A GIVEN AGE**

	30
20	
5		
50-70 years	70-79 years	80 and older
	AGE	

Figure 8-9

**SURVIVAL RATE IN PROSTATE CANCER ACCORDING TO
STAGE WITH OR WITHOUT TREATMENT**

	5 years	10 years	15 years
Stage 1	95-98%	85-90%	75-80%
Stage 2	70-80%	40-50%	15-25%
Stage 3	20%	5-10%	0-2 %

Figure 8-10

121

COMPLICATIONS OF RADICAL PROSTATECTOMY

1. **Total incontinence** - have no control of urination - 0 to 20%.

2. **Stress incontinence** - incontinence with coughing or lifting heavy objects - 30 to 60%

3. **Impotence** - 30% to 90% of patients may wait for a year for their potency to return

Note: The large variation in complication rates are due to changing techniques in performing the operation and because some surgeons underestimate their complication rates.

Figure 8-11

is performed. In Subclasses A2, B, and C a radical prostatectomy is sometimes recommended. This procedure involves the removal of the entire prostate gland and adjacent structures and, even in the best of hands, can be complicated by incontinence and impotence (Figure 8-11). Radiation therapy may be used in place of radical prostatectomy. Studies have shown it to be as effective as surgical treatment and to have fewer side effects. However, even radiation treatment causes impotence in 15% to 35% of cases. Another complication, colitis or inflammation of the colon, causes diarrhea and in rare cases, a colostomy is required.

In Stage 2 and Stage 3, no cure is possible, but treatment can greatly enhance patient comfort. Sometimes the tumor becomes so enlarged that the patient cannot urinate and surgery or radiation treatment is necessary. Bone pain from metastases may be reduced in selected patients by decreasing the male hormone, testosterone. This may be done by surgical castration or medical therapy. While castration is viscerally repulsive, the procedure is quick, relatively painless and effective. It is even possible to have artificial testes implanted for cosmetic reasons. There are medications that can simulate castration. Unlike breast cancer, though, patients often only respond once to hormonal therapy. Radiation therapy can also relieve pain, but chemotherapy is used infrequently in prostate cancer.

What I Would Do If I Had Prostate Cancer

Now that you are totally confused, let me tell you what I would do if I had prostate cancer. I would refuse all treatment with Stage 2 or Stage 3 disease if I was not in pain unless my urologist felt strongly that he could prevent complications from the tumor. If I developed a problem from the tumor itself, such as the inability to urinate, I would accept the treatment my urologist recommended. If I was in pain from the tumor, I would accept medical hormonal therapy. If this was ineffective I would try analgesics and regional nerve blocks. If this did not help, I would consent to radiation therapy if my physician thought it would be helpful.

With Stage 1 disease, I would follow the procedure that my urologist recommended to maximize a chance for a cure if I was under 70 years old. Although there is a reasonable possibility that surgical treatment could cause impotence and incontinence, I personally would prefer these complications to death. If the cancer recurred at a later time, I would accept treatment only for comfort and pain control. Between the ages of 70 to 80, I would be reluctant to accept surgery but would accept radiation treatment.

After 80, I would accept treatment for symptoms only. If my urologist strongly disagreed with my refusal of treatment, he would have to convince me that surgical treatment would have a strong chance of increasing my life span and give a strong incentive to risk being impotent and attired in diapers the rest of my life.

BRAIN CANCER

Brain tumors are among the most feared by patients, probably because they find their way onto television dramas. They can strike at a young age and every patient who complains to a doctor about headaches worries whether or not he has a brain tumor. There are a large variety of brain tumors. Unlike other cancers, there are strong data to suggest that aggressive treatment of malignant brain tumors increases survival and enhances the quality of life. However, they are still uniformly fatal.

Brain tumors are suspected in patients with headaches, mental status changes, seizures and vomiting. When the diagnosis is confirmed by a CAT scan or MRI, the doctor must determine whether the tumor is metastatic or "primary" — a tumor of the brain tissue itself — and if the tumor is benign or malignant. Another issue is whether the tumor is "operable" — accessible by the surgical techniques available (Figure 8-12). Tumors located deep in the brain can not be resected because too much damage is done to normal brain tissue. New techniques of computer-assisted surgery with microthin suction devices may soon render virtually all tumors operable.

Please look at Figure 8-13 which shows the distribution of the types of brain tumors in adults. A metastatic brain tumor often originates from lung cancer in males and breast cancer in females, although any type of cancer is possible. No cure is known but surgery, chemotherapy and radiation therapy may give an additional six months of life. Those who refuse all treatment generally succumb in two to three months.

The primary brain tumors shown in Figure 8-13 have a prognosis that is directly related to whether they are malignant and to the degree of malignancy. Pituitary tumors are rarely malignant and patients do fabulously well if the tumor is diagnosed before there is structural damage to the brain. Meningiomas, which are tumors of the lining that encases the brain, do respond to surgery and radiation treatment, although death invariably results if the tumor is malignant. Gliomas, which are tumors of the brain tissue, are more complex. Survival is dependent upon the DEGREE of malignancy, a determination that is made by pathologists. Gliomas are rated from Grade I to Grade IV, the latter being the most life-threatening (Figure 8-14).

```
┌─────────────────────────────────────────────────────┐
│                                                     │
│  MAJOR ISSUES IN TREATING BRAIN TUMORS              │
│                                                     │
│  1. Is the tumor primary or metastatic?             │
│  2. Is the tumor operable?                          │
│  3. Is the tumor benign or malignant?               │
│                                                     │
└─────────────────────────────────────────────────────┘
```

Figure 8-12

There are many complex protocols for the treatment of brain tumors. Most involve surgical resection followed by radiation therapy and/or chemotherapy. Sometimes, neurosurgeons will recommend a needle biopsy of a brain tumor before deciding the best course of action either to ascertain if the tumor is primary or metastatic, or because the tumor is inaccessible.

What I Would Do If I Had A Brain Tumor

My approach would depend upon my level of comfort. If I had a metastatic brain tumor and was entering the terminal phase (poor appetite, weight loss, etc.), I would not accept surgical treatment. I would consider radiation therapy if I had severe headaches or mental status changes. On the other hand, if I was able to function, I would consent to surgery if my neurosurgeon recommended it, fully aware that this, at best, would give me an additional several months of life.

With a primary brain tumor, I would accept aggressive surgical treatment hoping for a cure. If the pathology report showed that I had a highly malignant tumor such as a Grade III or Grade IV glioma, I would accept postoperative chemotherapy and radiation therapy as long as neither was causing debilitating side effects and I was able to enjoy life. If I saw that my condition was deteriorating rapidly, I would refuse all further treatment. If the tumor recurred, I would not consent to further surgery. With Grade I and Grade II tumors, I would follow the treatment recommended by my neurosurgeon and oncologist until I entered the terminal cancer phase, at which point I would refuse all non-comfort treatment.

TYPES OF BRAIN TUMORS SEEN IN ADULTS

Metastatic	50%
Primary	
Gliomas	25-30%
Meningiomas	10%
Pituitary	8%
Others	2-7%

Figure 8-13

SURVIVAL PERCENTAGE IN PRIMARY BRAIN TUMORS WITH TREATMENT

	6 months	1 year	5 years	10 years
Gliomas				
Grade I	98%	95%	50-95%*	40-90%*
Grade II	90%	80%	30%	10%
Grade III	50%	30%	10%	1-2%
Grade IV	60%	10%	0%	0%
Meningioma	95%	85%	75%	55%
Pituitary Tumor	98%	95%	90%	80%

*Survival rates in Grade I gliomas also depend on the location of the tumor

Figure 8-14

SURVIVAL IN COMMON DIGESTIVE TRACT TUMORS			
Tumor Type	Average Lifespan	1-Year Survival	5-Year Survival
Esophagus	5-7 months	35%	8%
Stomach	12-16 months	55%	17%
Pancreas	6 months	10%	3%
Liver	3-4 months	10%	4%

Figure 8-15

COMMON DIGESTIVE TRACT TUMORS (ESOPHAGUS, STOMACH, PANCREAS, LIVER)

Digestive tract tumors have a dismal prognosis (Figure 8-15). Pancreatic cancer killed Michael Landon within three months. Both of President Carter's siblings, Ruth Stapleton and Billy Carter were dead within a year of being so diagnosed.

In some cases, an attempt can be made to surgically remove the tumor. Before the patient agrees to embark on this route, both he and his physician should be convinced the tumor is not metastatic. The surgical procedures used in the frequently futile attempts to cure these poor patients are complicated, invasive, require an extensive recovery period and have a significant mortality rate. If surgery is unsuccessful and the tumor recurs, it is usually in the patient's best interests to accept further treatment for comfort only.

Chemotherapy and radiation therapy can sometimes be palliative, but have little effect on survival. Spinal anesthesia and infiltration of affected nerves may relieve pain. In esophageal cancer, the patient may be unable to swallow. Radiation treatment or the placement of a tube in the esophagus to bypass the tumor is often comforting.

What I Would Do If I Had a Digestive Tract Tumor

If my surgeon felt a surgical CURE was possible, I would accept surgery. Otherwise I would refuse all treatment unless I was in severe discomfort. I would then accept pain medications and spinal anesthesia. Only if they were unsuccessful would I try chemotherapy and/or radiation therapy. If I still was in severe pain, I would accept surgery if my surgeon honestly felt it might offer some relief.

KIDNEY (RENAL CELL) CANCER

Kidney cancer is common and usually presents with blood in the urine, weight loss or abdominal pain. Sometimes these tumors secrete hormones that cause bizarre seemingly-unrelated symptoms such as enlarged breasts in males or facial hair in females. These hormones may also cause high blood pressure and anemia.

Kidney cancer is staged as listed in Figure 8-16. Patients with distant metastases (Stage 4) are given the option of chemotherapy and those who respond (i.e. the tumors shrink in size) live longer than non-responders. Whether this is the result of the chemotherapy or simply because the tumors that respond are less malignant is unknown.

Notice in Figure 8-16 that a significant percentage, 11%, survive at least five years with metastatic disease. Radiation therapy may control pain in these patients when the tumor spreads to the bones. Surgery is sometimes advisable if the tumors are secreting hormones that are causing annoying and debilitating symptoms.

If the tumor is localized (Stage 1, 2 or 3) an attempt is made to cure the patient by removing the involved tumor. Fortunately, the patient's lifestyle is not affected because one kidney is adequate. The surgeon also biopsies the surrounding lymph nodes and if the pathologist finds any of them to be cancerous, the prognosis is worse.

What I Would Do If I Had Kidney Cancer

If I had kidney cancer without metastases (Stage 1, 2 or 3), I would allow my surgeon to attempt removal of the entire tumor with whatever technique she felt was most effective. If the tumor recurred after surgical removal, I would accept comfort treatment only. I would refuse all treatment with metastatic disease unless I was in pain and my physician felt radiation therapy or chemotherapy would help. If I had a metastatic tumor that was causing symptomatic hormonal imbalances, I would consent to surgery if medical treatments failed.

STAGING AND PROGNOSIS OF KIDNEY CANCER

	Definition	5-Year Survival
Stage 1	Tumor is confined to kidney	80%
Stage 2	Tumor invades sheath that surrounds kidney	65%
Stage 3	Tumor invades blood vessels that supply kidney	42%
Stage 4	Tumor is metastatic	11%

Figure 8-16

OVARIAN CANCER

Ovarian cancer is a diverse cancer and prognosis varies greatly depending not only on the stage but on the aggressiveness of the tumor. The vast majority of ovarian cancers are diagnosed after having metastasized and the common presenting symptoms of abdominal pain and bloating are caused by fluid secreted by the tumor(s) that have spread inside the abdomen. Rarely is a tumor that is still confined to an ovary large enough to cause symptoms. This is the tragedy of ovarian cancer.

Once suspected, a pelvic examination is done (most gynecologists do this routinely on their patients) and if a mass is felt, an ultrasound is performed. Sometimes a needle biopsy of the tumor can confirm the diagnosis, but most patients have a staging laparotomy (a surgical exploration of the abdomen) in which the ovaries, uterus and fallopian tubes are removed and multiple biopsies are performed. If large amounts of tumor are found in the layers of the internal organs, they are removed — "debulking." CAT scans and liver-spleen scans are done to see if the cancer has spread to distant organs. Based on the results, the patient is staged according to Figure 8-17. Pathologists further divide ovarian cancer into three grades, the first being the least aggressive and the third being the most. Sometimes pathologists are not even sure if tissue from an ovarian mass is malignant or not. The unfortunate patient is left in limbo.

Figure 8-18 illustrates the prognosis in ovarian cancer. In Stage 1 ovarian cancer, a surgical cure is possible. Some oncologists believe that radiation treatment administered postoperatively increases the cure rate. The treatment of metastatic ovarian cancer involves every permutation of most chemotherapeutic drugs ever invented, along with radiation therapy. Unlike most tumors discussed in this chapter, there are data to show that aggressive surgical treatment along with radiation therapy and chemotherapy can increase life span in metastatic disease (Stages 2, 3 and 4). Nonetheless, ovarian cancer is fatal unless it can be completely removed surgically.

SIMPLIFIED STAGING OF OVARIAN CANCER

Stage 1 tumor is limited to the ovaries

Stage 2 tumor extends into the pelvis

Stage 3 tumor extends into the lining of the abdomen

Stage 4 tumor is metastatic to a distant organ such as the liver

Figure 8-17

OVARIAN CANCER SURVIVAL IN TREATED PATIENTS

	5-Year Survival		5-Year Survival
Stage 1		**Stage 3**	
Grade 1	85%	Grade 1	45%
Grade 2	74%	Grade 2	15%
Grade 3	40%	Grade 3	8%
Stage 2		**Stage 4**	
Grade 1	57%	Grade 1	22%
Grade 2	50%	Grade 2	5%
Grade 3	45%	Grade 3	5%

Figure 8-18

What I Would Recommend If My Mother Had Ovarian Cancer

With Stage 1 disease, I would have her surgeon attempt a cure with the technique he felt gave her the best odds. In Stages 2, 3 and 4, I would have her consent to aggressive treatment including surgery, radiation therapy and chemotherapy with the hope that she would survive several additional years. When the tumor recurred, I would have her accept one more course of radiation therapy and/or chemotherapy but no more. If her surgeon felt debulking the tumor would be helpful, I would recommend she consent to the procedure one time. After this I would just see to it that she is kept comfortable.

ENDOMETRIAL (UTERINE) CANCER

Patients with endometrial cancer have a good prognosis because the most common symptom, inappropriate uterine bleeding, usually occurs before the cancer has spread. The gynecologist biopsies the suspicious areas and if the pathologist identifies endometrial cancer, a chest X-ray, bone scan and intravenous pyelogram (a test that studies the urinary system), are performed in search of metastatic disease.

Basically, though, staging is combined with the mainstay of therapy, a hysterectomy. While endometrial cancer is a disease usually found in post-menopausal women, modern surgical techniques have enabled cures for minimal endometrial cancers in young women who desire children. During the procedure, the surgeon looks to see if the tumor has spread to other structures. Biopsies of regional lymph nodes are performed. The pathologist examines these organs and determines the degree of malignancy of the tumor. Based on her findings, the patient is placed into a stage per Figure 8-19.

The treatment of endometrial cancer is in flux and a source of constant debate in the medical community. Patients with Stage 1 and 2 cancer are also given radiation treatment in addition to a hysterectomy. Those in which the tumor invades deeply into the uterus or whose cell types exhibit a high degree of malignancy are given higher radiation dosages to larger areas. Complicated radiation therapy protocols are used. If the cancer recurs, additional surgery and radiation may be given but there is no proof that these modalities prolong life. In Stage 3 and Stage 4, a surgical cure is not possible and the treatment is radiation and hormonal therapy. Those who respond to hormonal therapy have a much better prognosis (Figure 8-20).

What I Would Recommend If My Mother-In-Law Had Endometrial Cancer (I get along with my mother-in-law)

If the cancer was in Stage 1 or 2, I would recommend she at least have a hysterectomy and any other surgical and radiation treatment her gynecologist recommended. If the lymph node biopsies during the procedure revealed spread, then I would have her accept one session of radiation treatment but no more. If the tumor recurred at a later

---

**SIMPLIFIED STAGING OF ENDOMETRIAL CANCER
ALONG WITH PROGNOSIS**

	Location	10-year survival
Stage 1	tumor is only in the uterus	79%
Stage 2	tumor extends to the cervix	50%
Stage 3	tumor extends into the vagina and/or supporting structures	27%
Stage 4	tumor extends to bladder or rectum or has metastasized	9%

Figure 8-19

**SURVIVAL IN PATIENTS WITH ADVANCED (STAGE 3
OR 4) OR RECURRENT ENDOMETRIAL CANCER**

	1 year	2 years	5 years
Hormone responders	65%	55%	30%
Hormone non-responders	20%	5%	2%

Figure 8-20

date, I would have her accept only hormonal treatment. I would reserve additional radiation or surgical treatment to alleviate pain if her gynecologist thought it would help.

With Stage 3 or Stage 4 endometrial cancer, I would recommend she accept only hormonal therapy unless surgery or radiation therapy would enhance her comfort. Sometimes, endometrial cancer can bleed enough to cause a severe anemia. In this case, a hysterectomy or radiation treatment may be warranted, even if there is little if any chance for a cure.

CERVICAL CANCER

Cervical cancer is similar to endometrial cancer in that it usually presents as abnormal uterine bleeding and is eminently treatable. Patients can live with the disease for years and treatment can be curative in the early stages.

Cervical cancer is diagnosed when the patient has symptoms or by a routine screening test called a PAP test. After the pathologist confirms the diagnosis, the patient is staged by doing a metastatic work-up and a laparotomy if necessary.

The stages of cervical cancer are complex and an abbreviated schematic can be seen in Figure 8-21. Stage 1 and early Stage 2 cervical cancer is usually treated with surgery and/or radiation therapy, while the remaining stages are treated with radiation therapy. Stage 4 may be treated with chemotherapy, although many physicians question its efficacy. As cervical cancer often occurs among young women who desire children or who are pregnant when diagnosed, treatment regimens will vary greatly depending on the reproductive wishes of the patient. A discussion of this is beyond the scope of this book. Suffice it to say that new techniques of laser surgery and cyrosurgery have made cures possible without diminishing reproductive potential. If cervical cancer recurs after an attempted surgical cure, the prognosis is grave. The 1-year survival rate is 15% and 5-year survival rate is less than 5 percent.

What I Would Recommend for a Patient With Cervical Cancer

In stage 1, 2 or 3, accept aggressive treatment as prescribed by your gynecologist. In stage 4, refuse all treatment except for comfort. If the cancer recurs after radiation or surgical treatment, consider refusing all treatment except for comfort.

*   *   *

STAGING AND PROGNOSIS OF CERVICAL CANCER

	Location	5-Year Survival
Stage 1	Tumor is only in cervix	92%
Stage 2	Tumor spreads into vagina	75%
Stage 3	Tumor spreads into pelvis	40%
Stage 4	Tumor spreads beyond pelvis	14%

Figure 8-21

SUMMARY

In general, the best approach to the common cancers is to try for a surgical cure if the cancer has not spread to the lymph nodes or distant organs. Once a cancer has metastasized or recurred, curative treatment may be unrealistic and treatment is directed towards enhancing patient comfort and increasing life span without sacrificing quality of life. This is not always easy.

If you have cancer, discuss your situation with your physician. Each cancer is different but the type of cancer and its stage can be used to predict your prognosis. If there is no spread of the cancer, your doctor will probably recommend attempting a surgical cure. There are exceptions though. Elderly males with prostate cancer are often left untreated because the cancer progresses slowly. Once your tumor has metastasized, you must decide for yourself how aggressive you want your doctors to be. Chemotherapy and radiation therapy rarely prolong life but may enhance comfort. Analgesics and nerve blocks can relieve pain.

Once you enter the terminal phase of cancer, consider accepting treatment only to enhance comfort. Avoid being artificially fed. Your final days will be more dignified if you remain in your home or a hospice. If you are unable to avoid hospitalization, make sure you are DNR (do not resuscitate) and are not subject to uncomfortable and stressful procedures.

CHAPTER 9

AIDS

AIDS (Acquired Immune Deficiency Syndrome), unlike the other diseases discussed in this book, attacks early life – the average age of diagnosis being 36. Those afflicted are cheated and die young but the key point is they die. In medicine, knowledge is inversely proportional to verbiage. Nowhere is this more true than in AIDS. While a plethora of literature exists on the disease, there is little consensus on the definition of AIDS, the nature of the virus or the intricacies of the modes of spread. In spite of billions of dollars of research, little progress has been made against AIDS since it was first recognized in the early eighties. An effective vaccine has not even been developed. This is not to indict the dedicated physicians and scientists battling this plague, but to illustrate that this is a perplexing disease.

The AIDS virus, called HIV for human immunodeficiency virus, can be transmitted when the blood or semen of an infected individual enters another individual's body, usually by sexual activity, sharing a contaminated needle or from a blood transfusion. A distinction must be made between an AIDS-virus (HIV) carrier and AIDS itself. Many individuals who are positive for HIV have no symptoms, although the HIV can cause fever, weight loss, enlarged lymph nodes, diarrhea and even dementia – AIDS prodrome. However, AIDS is when the HIV attacks the immune system and allows the multitudes of microor-

---

SIMPLIFIED CLASSIFICATION OF HIV INFECTION

1. HIV carrier - HIV in the body without symptoms
2. AIDS prodrome - weight loss, fevers, diarrhea and swollen lymph glands (also called AIDS-related complex)
3. AIDS - at least one opportunistic infection or characteristic malignancy (definition has recently been extended to include a T4-cell count of less than 200)

Figure 9-1

COMMON AIDS-RELATED INFECTIONS AND CANCERS

Toxoplasmosis	Kaposi's Sarcoma
Cryptococcus	Lymphoma
Pneumocystis	Candida
Cytomegalovirus	Histoplasmosis
Tuberculosis	

Figure 9-2

ganisms that surround us to cause potentially-deadly diseases — opportunistic infections (Figure 9-1). This weakened immune system also predisposes AIDS patients to certain types of cancers. Thus, AIDS is when an HIV carrier contracts an opportunistic infection or a characteristic malignancy (Figure 9-2).

Once the HIV invades the body, it attacks several types of cells, but the important one is called the T-helper cell (T4), a major player in the infinitely-complex immune system. When enough T-helper cells are rendered impotent by the AIDS virus, the victim's immune system malfunctions and the patient contracts an opportunistic infection — AIDS. This can take anywhere from months to over a decade, the

PROBABILITY OF DEVELOPING AIDS IN A GIVEN
AMOUNT OF YEARS AFTER DIAGNOSED AS HIV
POSITIVE*

Years	Probability	Years	Probability
1	0.2%	9	60%
2	1.0%	10	70%
3	3.0%	11	80%
4	11%	12	85%
5	20%	13	90%
6	33%	14	95%
7	40%	15	99%
8	50%		

* Note that these data were accumulated before the FDA changed the
definition of AIDS to include those with T4-cell counts of less than 200.

Figure 9-3

average being eight years. Please look at Figure 9-3 which gives the
probability of developing AIDS each year after the initial HIV infection. Notice that less than 1 percent of those infected with HIV develop
AIDS within two years, whereas it is estimated that 99% will develop
AIDS within 15 years. Thus, those who developed AIDS in the early
1980's were the unlucky ones who happened to develop opportunistic
infections quickly. Needless to say, this has ominous implications as
many infections occurred in the early 1980's before education altered
the behavior patterns in some individuals.

Thus, many HIV-positive individuals will remain symptom-free for
years and often for a decade. Is there anyway to know if developing
AIDS is imminent? Not with complete certainty but laboratory tests
can give some clues. As would be expected, the T4-cell count is a good
predictor as a deficiency in this cell type is the cause of a malfunctioning
immune system. Please refer to Figure 9-4. As you can see, the
concentration of T4 cells in the blood correlates to the chance of getting
AIDS in the near future. A patient with a T4-cell count of less than

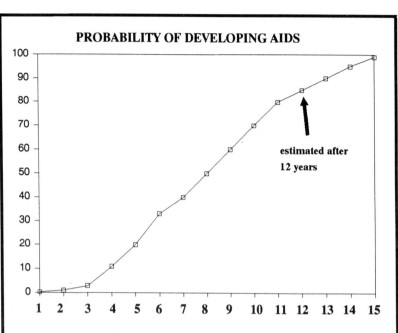

PROBABILITY OF DEVELOPING AIDS

estimated after
12 years

How to read this chart - The table and the graph represent the same information. For example, a man who was diagnosed as HIV-positive today has a 3 percent chance of developing AIDS within three years and a 50% chance of developing AIDS within eight years. Notice that the last several years are estimates because the disease has not been studied for 15 years.

Figure 9-3 (continued)

100 has about a 60% chance of developing AIDS within a year-and-a-half. As a matter of fact, the Federal Disease Center has revised the definition of AIDS to include an individual who has a T4-cell count of 200 or lower, even if he has never had an opportunistic infection. Other tests that enable your doctor to assess your risk are the Beta-2 micro-globulin and p24 antigen, both of which increase prior to the onset of opportunistic infections.

PROBABILITY OF DEVELOPING AIDS BASED ON THE T4 COUNT*

T4 count	% developing AIDS (old definition) within 18 months
100	60%
200	35%
300	15%
400	10 %
500	5%

*AIDS being defined as the onset of an opportunistic infection or characteristic malignancy

Figure 9-4

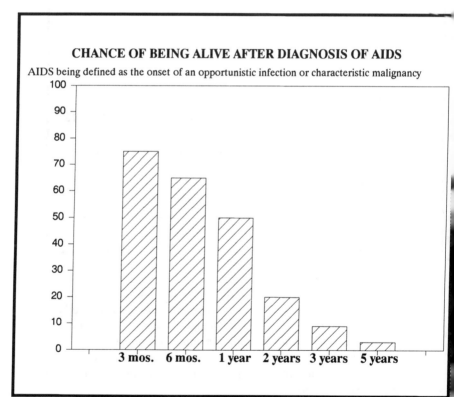

CHANCE OF BEING ALIVE AFTER DIAGNOSIS OF AIDS

AIDS being defined as the onset of an opportunistic infection or characteristic malignancy

Figure 9-5

AVERAGE SURVIVAL TIME OF AIDS VICTIMS

Initial Presentation	Survival Time
Kaposi's Sarcoma	21 months
Pneumocystis Pneumonia (1984)	10 months
Pneumocystis Pneumonia (1990)*	17 months
Other opportunistic infections	10 months

*better treatment has improved survival in Pneumocystis pneumonia

Figure 9-6

Once a patient develops AIDS, death is inevitable. At present, the longest an AIDS patient has survived is eight years. While there is some evidence that superior health care can prolong life, the fortunate few that live for several years do so primarily because they have a disease that progresses at a slower rate, not because of brilliant interventions by the medical profession. Please look at Figure 9-5. Fifty percent of AIDS victims are dead one year after the diagnosis and 25% die within three months.

The expected life span of an AIDS victim varies, depending on the disease's initial manifestations. For example, a patient whose first manifestation of AIDS is Kaposi's sarcoma, a type of lymphatic cancer, lives for an average of 21 months. On the other hand, those who present with Pneumocystis pneumonia only survive 10 months although this has increased with improved treatment (Figure 9-6).

I do not mean to overwhelm you with statistics but it is important that AIDS victims understand that the medical community is abysmally ignorant of AIDS and that aggressively pursuing the treatment of an opportunistic infection will not significantly enhance an AIDS victim's survival unless the patient has Pneumocystis pneumonia. As can be seen in Figure 9-6, the average survival in this subclass of patients has increased from 10 months in 1984 to 17 months in 1990.

However, those who opt for aggressive treatment should understand the ramifications of their decision. Even if treatment eliminates the Pneumocystis pneumonia, another hideous complication is lurking around the corner. Endstage AIDS is not pleasant. Recurrent infections attack every organ system. Weak patients with intractable diarrhea soil themselves. As with other terminal diseases, mundane chores — cleaning, cooking, bathing, shopping — become impossible. Patients can look forward to rampant fevers, depression and dementia. Rapid weight loss and eye infections may result in a pox-covered blind human skeleton with contracted limbs and cavitous bedsores. Those of you who have seen an AIDS victim die know that my characterization is not fictionalized.

Doctors treating AIDS victims often feel obligated to perform multiple tests. Most doctors are uncomfortable rendering treatment without a diagnosis. It is counter to everything they learned in medical school and instills tremendous feelings of insecurity and incompetence. Doctors are compulsive people who like to be in control. Thus AIDS victims find themselves subject to inconvenient, unpleasant and painful procedures such as endoscopies, biopsies and spinal taps. Medications used in AIDS patients have numerous side effects such as nausea and vomiting. In medieval times, gays were tortured to save their souls. In twentieth-century America, they are tortured to save their bodies.

Many AIDS victims accept treatment and then later become hostile towards the medical establishment when it is unsuccessful and feel like guinea pigs. If you have AIDS, only you can decide how much treatment you are willing to endure. Do not delude yourself into thinking that a cure is around the corner. It isn't. Our comprehension of the immune system is comparable to Saddam Hussein's understanding of human rights. During medical school, in the middle of an arcane discussion of null cells, T-helper cells and opsonins, my immunology professor turned towards the class and said, "You realize that half of what I am teaching you is wrong, but I do not know which half it is."

I hate to be overly pessimistic, but if you have AIDS, please do not pounce on every new discovery than comes out on a weekly basis. These "breakthroughs" are often a function of medical politics and to increase the profit margins of speculators in drug company stocks.

In 1984, I worked as a physician in Haiti and cared for many AIDS victims. In my book, *The Neglected and Abused*, I wrote the following:

"Nobody bothered Andre [an AIDS victim with cytomelaglovirus in his eyes] and he lived for three weeks, comfortably and pain free until he quietly passed away in his sleep. In a sense, Andre was lucky to be in Haiti. In the United States, he would have been subject to a variety of tortures of which even the most imaginative fire-and-brimstone preacher could not conceive. Even a member of the Moral Majority, who concluded AIDS was God's revenge for wayward behavior, would wince when he saw what AIDS victims endured during attempts to cure them.

In the United States, Andre would have had multiple spinal taps, skin biopsies, lung biopsies, tubes up his rectum, tubes down his throat, tubes down his nose, tubes in his penis, needles in his arteries, needles in his veins, needles in his eyes and spears in his bones. He would have taken drugs that made him vomit bile, lose his hair, made him dizzy, burned his skin and destroyed his kidneys. He would have had CAT scans, liver scans, kidney scans and bone scans. He would have been inundated with internists, proctologists, oncologists, ophthalmologists, hematologists, neurologists, dermatologists, pulmonologists and nephrologists, all ordering different tests to justify their consultation. After being harassed by residents, tortured by interns and bored by social workers, he would have still died. Andre was much better off in Haiti."

TREATMENT

Now that the reader is aware of my bias on the treatment of AIDS, permit me to review some of the options available. To write an exhaustive analysis of present-day AIDS treatment would require a larger book. Thus I will confine myself to common infections and problems. Basically there are two kinds of treatment — one that directly attacks the HIV and another that attacks opportunistic infections. Some opportunistic infections can be palliated and others cannot.

DIRECT ATTACK OF HIV

The major treatment that actually attacks HIV is AZT (Azidothymidine, Zidovudine, Retrovir) which is being given in patients who have AIDS or are HIV-positive. In HIV-carriers, it delays the onset of AIDS. In some studies, AZT has also been found to increase life span in those with AIDS by one year.

There is still debate as to whether or not AZT is effective. When AZT was first discovered, researchers did not realize that many patients positive for HIV could live for years without developing AIDS. Five to ten years from now, it may be discovered that those who did well on AZT were simply patients whose disease progressed in a less virulent fashion. It has also been noted that AZT is less effective in AIDS patients who continue to reexpose themselves to the HIV by persisting in high-risk behavior such as unsafe sex and the use of intravenous drugs. Those willing to comply with AZT treatment may simply be the same patients who changed their behavior and avoided further dosages of HIV.

AZT can have nasty side effects such as an anemia that requires periodic transfusions and medications to stimulate the bone marrow to produce more red blood cells. AZT may also cause nausea and muscle pain that must be treated with other medications. In some patients, it even makes the eyelashes grow longer.

Whether patients who take AZT live longer because of the drug or because of lifestyle changes may never be known. In any case, it would be foolish not to avail oneself of a medication that may give an additional year of life.

TREATMENT OF OPPORTUNISTIC INFECTIONS

Pneumocystis Pneumonia

Lung involvement is common in AIDS and the most frequent infection is Pneumocystis Carinii pneumonia (PCP), occurring in over 40% of patients. Diagnosing Pneumocystis pneumonia can be a long and painful ordeal of blood cultures, sputum specimens, X-rays and lung biopsies, but treatment is highly effective. The problem is that recurrence is common. Maintenance medications, Bactrim and Pentamidine, have an annual cost of $3,000-$4,000. Patients with severe Pneumocystis pneumonia who must be placed on respirators have a dismal prognosis, an 85% mortality rate. The few survivors do poorly and are almost always dead within a year.

Infections and Cancers of the Brain

Infections and cancers of the brain are the most feared complications in AIDS because they can steal the patient's ability to think and reason. Forty percent to 80% of AIDS victims develop irreversible mental dysfunction from one of three things:

1. Direct brain infection by the AIDS virus (HIV)
2. Opportunistic infections of the brain
3. Brain cancers

The direct brain infection by HIV is called AIDS-dementia complex (ADC). Initial symptoms are poor concentration, social withdrawl and forgetfulness, followed by progression to complete dementia. Even patients who appear to be functioning normally show slight mental impairments when checked with mental function tests that assess abstract reasoning and memory. The tragic aspect of this entity is that it may present before the patient has AIDS. Remember, this is a direct attack on the brain cells by the HIV, not an opportunistic infection. Thus, patients with ADC may live a long time. AZT has shown some promise in slowing the progression of ADC but does not reverse the initial damage.

Unlike ADC, patients with opportunistic brain infections and brain cancers do not typically become demented. Rather they have specific symptoms such as seizures, headaches, paralysis or the inability to remember names. These infections may respond to treatment, but can return with a vengence. Often it is difficult for doctors to diagnose the type of infection. CAT scans and MRI's may leave more questions than answers and patients must undergo a spinal tap, an unpleasant procedure in which a long needle is placed between the bones encasing the spinal cord while the apprehensive patient lies in a fetal position. Sometimes the only way to diagnose the cause is by performing a brain biopsy. Even when a cause is found, the treatments have considerable side effects, but two specific entities do occasionally respond: crypto-coccal meningitis and toxoplasmosis.

Cryptococcal meningitis is treated with a drug called Amophotericin-B which is nicknamed by physicians as "Amphoterrible" because of its numerous side effects. A recent drug, Fluconazole, can be given orally. The infection may regress but, it is never eradicated so the patient must be on medication for the rest of his life. Toxoplasmosis is treated with two powerful drugs, sulfadiazine and pyrethamine, neither of which eradicate the infection but can control it. Some doctors insist on multiple tests including a brain biopsy before initiating treatment of these infections while others are happy to try the medications empirically and see if the patient's condition improves. This can save the patient a lot of grief. Often patients have permanent brain damage and must be placed in a nursing home or hospice.

Brain cancers in AIDS patients are usually lymphomas. Lyle Alzado had the same type of brain lymphoma seen in AIDS victims although in his case, it was supposedly due to immune suppression caused by steroids. Brain lymphomas typically occur towards the end of an AIDS patient's life. He is usually treated with radiation but some new chemotherapeutic regimens are being also devised. Neither modality has been proven to prolong life.

Weight loss

Weight loss is seen in all AIDS patients and becomes precipitous at the endstage of the disease. It is due either to poor appetite or because of diarrhea caused by the inability of the intestines to absorb nutrition. Patients have to use their judgement in deciding how aggressive they want their doctors to be. Diarrhea may be due to a treatable infection or from lymphoma and Kaposi's sarcoma of the intestines, entities in which treatment is of dubious efficacy.

A general lack of appetite is a more difficult problem. Unless the patient is acutely ill, a poor appetite signifies that death is inevitable. Unless these patients assert themselves, they will be attacked with tube feedings and intravenous nutrition, neither of which has been shown to prolong life. Pharmacies and laboratories are big money makers in hospitals and often compensate for lost revenues in outpatient and emergency room departments. Between high-priced solutions, sophisticated intravenous catheters and requisite laboratory studies, a patient on artificial nutrition can generate $1,500 in fees a day. There is nothing sadder than an AIDS patient who pulls out his feeding tube while bevies of social workers and psychiatrists try to figure out why he is refusing to be tortured.

Blindness

AIDS patients often go blind, usually from cytomegalovirus or fungal infections. The medical literature is replete with studies on how to treat these infections and there is no consensus of opinion. Treatment involves intravenous medications and surgery. While treatment sometimes helps, cases often clear up spontaneously leading to speculation that treatment does not alter the natural course of the disease. On the other hand, many studies have shown that treatment can prevent infections from spreading to the other eye when only one eye is involved. Blind patients with AIDS only live a matter of months.

FINANCIAL AND LEGAL ASPECTS IN DEALING WITH AIDS

The blunt reality is that insurance companies acted swiftly and effectively in limiting their liability in paying the health care costs of AIDS victims. Every year a higher percentage of AIDS victims are forced to rely on public assistance. Many AIDS victims are lulled into believing that some anti-discrimination statute will prevent insurance companies from denying coverage. Insurance companies are good at excluding high-risk populations from their rolls without overt discrimination. When I finished my residency in New York City, I lived in Manhattan's East Village. I found it impossible to obtain health insurance even though I was a fiscally-responsible physician and engaged to be married. I later discovered that my zip code, 10003, was a red flag for the insurance companies. In another instance, a patient of mine who owns a hair dressing salon confided to me that obtaining health coverage for her employees was impossible. All her employees were female. I told her to explicitly state this in her next application, and miraculously, health insurance was extended to her business. Many AIDS victims feel they will be able to fight discrimination.

COMPARISON OF PAYMENTS OF PRIVATE INSURANCE
VERSUS MEDICAID (1991)

	Medicaid	Private Insurance
New York		
Office Visit	$24	$60
Hospital Visit	$24	$60
San Francisco		
Office Visit	$18	$50
Hospital Visit	$28	$65

Figure 9-7

Unfortunately, AIDS is so debilitating and draining that it is hard to sustain a prolonged fight. The insurance companies know this. On the other hand, being on public assistance is not always a terrible thing. Much publicity has been generated to imply that uninsured AIDS patients receive inferior care. The opposite is true. The first biopsy done on an AIDS patient is a wallet biopsy. Thus, insured patients are often given lucrative but ineffective and painful treatments. For example, if an AIDS patient is admitted to a hospital with a brain lymphoma, he is going to die whether he is treated or not. Perhaps treatment will give him several more weeks, but not pleasant ones. A patient on Medicaid may not be treated because the reimbursement for the radiation treatments and artificial feedings will be so poor that the hospital will lose money. On the other hand, a patient with good private insurance may be given aggressive and futile care.

This does not mean that you should drop your private health insurance if you have AIDS. While it is easy for you to qualify for Medicaid, it greatly limits your freedom in choosing doctors and exercising your health care options. Medicaid reimburses doctors and hospitals very unsatisfactorily (Figure 9-7). Since chronic budget deficits are plaguing the state and federal governments, these governments subject doctors who care for Medicaid patients to periodic audits and constant harassment in a feeble attempt to control costs. Thus, private physicians often refuse to care for Medicaid patients. You must either go to clinics where the time spent with your physician is measured in seconds, or camp out in the emergency room of a public hospital where you will be preempted by asthma attacks, drug overdoses and gun-shot wounds before being seen by a doctor eight hours after your arrival. If you need to be admitted, you may lie on a stretcher in the emergency room for days until a bed becomes available. Also, private insurance often reimburses better for hospice and home care, both of which are crucial for AIDS victims. Your interests are better served if you have private insurance and assert yourself when you do desire treatment.

AIDS and those with disabling ARC (AIDS-related complex) may qualify for disability and therefore be eligible for Medicare which reimburses doctors and other health care workers at higher rates than Medicaid. The problem is that the requirements to qualify for disability are vague and many AIDS victims are too incapacitated to deal with the bureaucracy. While much ballyhoo is made about the large AIDS budget, a large portion goes to fund research rather than providing benefits for the victims. HIV-carriers and AIDS patients must plan carefully if their final days are to have a modicum of dignity. A good reference on the benefits and rights of AIDS patients is:

The AIDS Benefit Handbook
by Thomas P. McCormick
Yale University Press

GENERAL RECOMMENDATIONS

1. Determine if AIDS is imminent if you are an HIV-carrier. Ask your doctor to perform the blood tests to see if you will develop AIDS in the near future. In the meantime, start saving money so that you will be able to maintain your health insurance when you are incapacitated and unable to work. Under no circumstances should you cancel your health insurance. While those with health insurance often receive aggressive and futile care, you have the option to refuse such care and are therefore in control.

149

2. Get your affairs in order. Make out a will. Do not delay because AIDS-dementia complex (ADC) can render you incapable of making rational decisions. If you write a will after a documented mental function disorder and you also have significant financial assets, it may be contested, even by family members who rejected you while you were alive. If you have a companion but die intestate (without a will), your companion has little if any legal claim to your estate. Remember, if you do not have any children, your estate goes to your parents in most states. While legal challenges may be possible, your companion may also become ill and not have the stamina to fight. Consider getting the two references below.

Wills Give You Power
The National Gay Rights Advocates
540 Castro Street
San Francisco, CA 94114
415-863-3624

Getting Your Affairs in Order
San Francisco AIDS Foundation
333 Valencia St.
San Francisco, CA 94103
415-861-3397

3. Choose a health care proxy. This can be a family member or a companion. While choosing your companion may seem logical, keep several factors in mind. Your companion may also have AIDS and may not be available when you are incapacitated. Often, a family member is a better choice. Many AIDS victims with gay lifestyles have had acrimonious experiences with their family. If possible, bury the hatchet. If you do not have a loyal companion, your family may care for you in your final days. Many AIDS victims die homeless and alone.

4. Once you are diagnosed with AIDS, sit down and discuss your prognosis with your doctor and formulate in your own mind how you desire to be treated. Stay away from high-powered academic physicians. Find a doctor who treats patients himself and is not fol-

lowed by a retinue of fawning residents and interns. Remember, while doctors have high-tech instrumentation at their finger tips, they do not have crystal balls. Do not expect clear-cut answers to your health care questions. Many AIDS victims are angry at society and vent this on their doctors. When doctors are forced to deal with angry patients, not only do they find it unpleasant, but they are wary of being sued.

5. Avoid charlatans. There are some people who profit from the misery of others. There are no treatments to stimulate the immune system. If someone wants you to try their vitamins, exercises or mantras — fine — but don't give anyone large amounts of money. There is no evidence that megadoses of any mineral or vitamin help AIDS patients.

6. If you are in the hospital, make sure you are a DNR (do not resuscitate). This does not mean no care, just no CPR (cardiopulmonary resuscitation). AIDS patients who are sick enough to require CPR rarely, if ever, survive to be discharged from the hospital. Even if you are given CPR, hospital personnel are reluctant to act aggressively as needle sticks and similar injuries to hospital personnel usually occur during the excitement of CPR.

7. Use common sense with regard to artificial feeding. If you can't eat because it hurts to swallow, your esophagus is obstructed or you have treatable diarrhea — accept artificial feeding. Remember that bowel lymphomas and Kaposi's sarcoma of the intestines are often refractory to treatment. Thus, artificial feedings will be of little benefit in these instances. If you simply have no appetite or you are demented, your body is telling you something — refuse artificial feedings. The human body rebels when forced to eat and death is held in abeyance for weeks at the most.

8. Once you reach a point where death is imminent, stay away from hospitals and emergency rooms. Poor prognostic signs are:

- rapid weight loss
- blindness
- dementia
- brain infections and brain cancers

Home care and hospice care is infinitely preferable to being hospitalized. You may even have a permanent intravenous line placed so that a home-health-care nurse can give you pain and comfort medications. Even if your private insurance carrier technically does not cover home care, give the insurance company a call. Home care and hospices average $50 to $200 a day whereas the care of a hospitalized AIDS patient can average over $1,000 a day. AIDS patients often stay in hospitals for months because they have nowhere to go. Just because you refuse aggressive treatment does not mean you do not have the right to decent, compassionate care.

WHAT I WOULD DO IF I HAD AIDS

If I found out I was HIV-positive, I would ask my doctor to routinely perform the appropriate tests (T4-cell count, p24 antigen, Beta-2 microglobulin) so that I could anticipate the onset of AIDS. I would accept AZT treatment if my physician recommended it.

Once AIDS developed, I would allow the doctors to treat my first infection aggressively but insist on being DNR meaning no intubation or CPR. I would continue with AZT treatment and maintenance medications as my physician recommended. For any brain infection, I would refuse treatment, although as alluded to earlier, toxoplasmosis and crytococcus often respond to treatment. If I had AIDS-dementia complex, I would refuse all treatment. My fear would be that I would have permanent brain damage and rendered mentally incompetent.

When I entered the terminal phase of AIDS, I would arrange hospice care or home care for myself and not permit myself to be admitted to a hospital unless I was in severe pain. I would not accept artificial feedings unless I had an appetite but was unable to swallow. I would accept no surgery unless it was to relieve pain or due to an unrelated condition, such as appendicitis.

CHAPTER 10

POSSIBLE SCENARIOS

Below are some typical situations that I have created to reinforce the main concepts in this book. Previously, situations have been discussed as if there is only one health problem. In actuality, this is rarely the case. Patients often have to make decisions based on multiple illnesses and must consider financial factors as well.

Case #1: Alzheimer's Disease

Mr. Cromwell is an 80-year-old who retired from a middle-management position in a major corporation at the age of 62. He and his wife live in suburban Philadelphia and spend their time visiting their children. He notices that he gets lost while driving in his own neighborhood and has had to ask gas station attendants for directions. He starts to avoid playing pinochle with has grandchildren because he cannot remember the rules of the game. Finally, at his wife's insistence, he sees his internist who says "these things happen when you get old" and refers him to a neurologist. A young crackerjack, the neurologist performs every conceivable test – a CAT scan, a MRI, a spinal tap and extracts more blood than Mr. Cromwell thought was in his body. All these tests have normal results. The neurologist refers Mr. Cromwell

153

to a psychiatrist who tests his short-term memory and judgement. Based on these findings, it is concluded that Mr. Cromwell has early Alzheimer's, there is no effective treatment and that his condition will continue to deteriorate.

Mr. and Mrs. Cromwell conclude their physicians are insensitive oafs, but draw up a living will and assign Mrs. Cromwell as Mr. Cromwell's health care proxy. During the next three years, Mr. Cromwell becomes increasingly frustrated by his inability to function and becomes belligerent when his wife refuses to give him the car keys. He becomes incontinent and Mrs. Cromwell is not strong enough to physically take him to the commode and clean him. She now realizes that his condition will only get worse, that institutionalization is inevitable and that it is going to cost money.

Mrs. Cromwell sits down with her accountant to assess their finances. Their house is worth $200,000 and although it is paid for, the upkeep and taxes are outrageously expensive. Their portfolio is worth $150,000, mostly in the stock of the corporation that employed Mr. Cromwell. The dividends from this, combined with their social security and pension have enabled them to live comfortably. The Cromwells must "spend down" before Medicaid will pay for his nursing home care. Many nursing homes refuse to take Mr. Cromwell because he has Alzheimer's. Mrs. Cromwell eventually finds a home at the cost of $5,500 a month. She is permitted to keep her house and $66,480 dollars, but the rest of their assets is spent on her husband's nursing home care.

While in the nursing home, a routine blood-screening reveals Mr. Cromwell to have anemia and a subsequent work-up reveals that he has colon cancer. Mr. Cromwell now is totally confused, recognizes only his wife and must be spoon-fed. Mrs. Cromwell refuses all treatment although the physician points out that the cancer may be curable with surgery. Meanwhile, Mr. Cromwell becomes impossible to feed and the physician informs Mrs. Cromwell that without a feeding tube, Mr. Cromwell will slowly starve. Again, Mrs. Cromwell refuses to allow a feeding tube. Mr. Cromwell then develops pneumonia and the physician recommends hospitalization for high-dose intravenous antibiotics. While Mr. Cromwell's breathing is labored, he is not in any obvious pain. Mrs. Cromwell refuses hospitalization and Mr. Cromwell passes away several days later.

Comment: The Cromwells may have been able to avoid losing a large portion of their portfolio with "clever" financial planning that would have entailed transferring a large portion of their assets to their children when Mr. Cromwell's Alzheimer's Disease was diagnosed. (Remember, assets must be transferred 30 months prior to becoming eligible for Medicaid). On the other hand, Mrs. Cromwell would not have had the freedom to choose the nursing home that best suited her husband's needs unless her children agreed to help pay. Also note that Mr. Cromwell may have lived several years longer if Mrs. Cromwell had consented to the surgical treatment of his colon cancer and hospitalization for pneumonia. While being Mr. Cromwell's health care proxy gave her the legal stature to refuse treatment, most doctors would have respected her wishes without her being a health care proxy as long as they were not being blamed by another family member for "allowing Dad to die."

Case #2 : Coma after a stroke

Mr. Austin is a 70-year-old retiree living in Texas, who has mild hypertension. While eating breakfast, he becomes confused and then falls out of his chair. Mr. Austin is taken by ambulance to the hospital where he becomes non-responsive and is intubated by the emergency room physician. A CAT scan shows a massive stoke.

A neurologist examines him and informs Mrs. Austin that her husband's chances are poor, but that he has seen rare cases where patients in his condition recover. Mr. Austin is treated aggressively and a nasogastric tube is placed for feeding. Over the next several days, Mr. Austin remains in a coma and several EEG's show minimal but definite brain activity. Mrs. Austin becomes increasingly frustrated at the inactivity on the part of the doctors and the deterioration of her husband of 50 years. Mr. Austin has a bout of pneumonia that is treated aggressively. After four weeks, the neurologist concludes that there is no reasonable hope for recovery and recommends turning off the respirator. Mrs. Austin refuses to accept this and requests a second opinion from another neurologist. The second neurologist concurs with the opinion of the first one and after another week of emotional agony and consultation with her minister and children, Mrs. Austin agrees. When the respirator is removed, Mr. Austin expires in a matter of minutes.

Comment: Although the Austins did not have living wills or health care proxies, the doctors were reluctant to turn off the respirator until Mrs. Austin gave her consent to do so. Also note that while Mr. Austin never technically fit the definition of brain death, his age and the length of his coma (over a month) made his chances for recovery virtually nil.

Case #3: Survival after a stroke

Mrs. Boyd is a diabetic 75-year-old woman who is active in community and church affairs. One day, her husband notices that her speech is garbled and takes her to the emergency room where she is diagnosed as having an evolving stroke and is admitted to the hospital. Two days later, Mrs. Boyd is paralyzed on her right side and when she attempts to speak, only gibberish comes out of her mouth. She remains mentally alert, understands everything that is said to her and is still able to read. After several days, she is discharged from the hospital but returns to the physical therapy department three times a week. As she is highly motivated, she learns to walk with a walker but even with intense speech therapy, she can only manage to say a few words.

In spite of her stroke, Mrs. Boyd remains upbeat. Although unable to write, she continues to make financial decisions and enjoys reading and watching television. When her vision diminishes, she consents to cataract surgery to restore it. Her main problem is bathing herself, using the bathroom and getting Mr. Boyd to cook a palatable meal. With the help of a social worker, Mrs. Boyd is able to obtain assistance in keeping her house clean for minimal cost. Meals-on-Wheels brings at least one good meal a day. Medicare partially funds home care to help with her insulin injections. When she falls and breaks her hip, she consents to aggressive surgical treatment and battles with a vicious bout of postoperative pneumonia. Later that year, she has a heart attack but recovers and returns to her house in good spirits where she continues to enjoy life. Her friends and grandchildren visit and she keeps up with Danielle Steel and Sidney Sheldon novels.

Comment: Mrs. Boyd has a strong will to live. Even with her multiple medical problems, Mrs. Boyd may live for many years. As long as she is enjoying life, she should continue to accept medical treatment. Patients like this are quite common.

Case #4 : Survival after a stroke

Mr. Taylor is a widowed 88-year-old who lives in a complex for senior citizens. Although he has always lived frugally, he worked as a manual laborer and never made a high salary. Poor financial decisions diminished his savings and now his only income is his social security check. Nonetheless, he enjoys watching television, especially the Boston Red Sox games and looks back with bemused satisfaction at all his friends who were more successful, but are now dead.

One day, he loses his sense of balance and the next thing he knows, he wakes up in a hospital bed surrounded by somber-looking men in white coats. One of them intones that he has had a stroke. When Mr. Taylor tries to reply, only grunts come out of his mouth. Another doctor informs him that the stroke has stolen his ability to speak and walk but with a little luck, these functions may return. They don't. The senior complex where he lived is not equipped to handle someone requiring his level of care. As he has no assets, the social worker petitions the state and he receives Medicaid. He is then placed in a nursing home.

Mr. Taylor considers this to be a fate worse than death. He is bound to a wheel chair, and dependent on attendants to feed and bathe him. He must push a buzzer everytime he has to go to the bathroom and if the attendants are slow, he soils himself. Mr. Taylor wants to die. Fortunately for him, the doctor assigned to him in the nursing home realizes this. When he contracts pneumonia, his doctor gives him the option of going to the hospital for aggressive treatment or remaining in the nursing home. Mr. Taylor refuses to go to the hospital and several days later, passes away.

Comment: Mr. Taylor's decision is entirely reasonable. Unlike the previous case, he did not have financial and social support. This diminished his will to live.

Case #5: Coronary Artery Disease

Mr. Baldwin is a 48-year-old high school teacher with a strong history of heart disease in his family. His father died at the age of 52 and both of his brothers have had bypass surgery. While jogging, he feels tightness in his chest and immediately goes to the emergency room where the decision is made to admit him to the hospital to rule out a heart attack. After several days, all the test results indicate he has not had a heart attack. His cardiologist performs a stress test and sees signs of coronary artery disease. Mr. Baldwin is given nitroglycerin tablets in the event the chest pain returns. For the next several years, Mr. Baldwin has occasional chest pain but becomes alarmed when he is unable to even play a round of golf without taking several pills. His cardiologist performs a cardiac catheterization that demonstrates large blockages of his coronary arteries. Surgery is recommended and Mr. Baldwin consents. Within several months, Mr. Baldwin is once again playing golf and jogging without chest pain.

Five years later, Mr. Baldwin has a prolonged episode of chest pain and his EKG in the emergency room shows a fresh heart attack. He is admitted to the hospital and a repeat cardiac catheterization demonstrates that his coronary arteries have reoccluded. Attempts to diminish his recurring chest pain with medication fail. Thus, repeat bypass surgery is recommended and Mr. Baldwin consents. He does well and a postoperative scan of his heart shows that his ejection fraction is 45%. Mr. Baldwin notes that he no longer has the same energy as before his heart attack and repeat surgery, but he is still able to teach and make a living. Two years later, he suffers another heart attack and this time, he is not as fortunate. His recovery is complicated by two episodes of congestive heart failure. A scan of his heart shows his ejection fraction to be only 22%.

Mr. Baldwin returns to his home but is no longer able to walk up a flight of stairs. Returning to his teaching position is out of the question. His cardiologist places him on digoxin, a diuretic and an afterload reducer. Nonetheless, Mr. Baldwin on several occasions, becomes short of breath and has to be admitted to the hospital to rid his lungs of fluid. Each episode of heart failure is worse than before, and Mr. Baldwin knows there is little his doctors can do to help, even though he is a young man of 55. He refuses further hospitalization and succumbs in his sleep several months later.

Comment: This case illustrates that coronary heart disease is a long-term disease unless the patient develops heart failure. Mr. Baldwin accepted state-of-the-art technology until he was unable to function. He remained coherent throughout his entire illness so that he was able to make rational decisions about his care.

Case #6 : COPD

Ms. Harrington is a 52-year-old advertising executive who has smoked since she was 13. She finds it ironic that she now has to sneak into the lavatory for a cigarette in her "smoke free" work environment, just as she had to in high school.

She was diagnosed as having COPD ten years ago. She had tried to stop smoking numerous times only to gain weight. She became so irritable that she blamed her second divorce on the insistence of her physician that she stop smoking. After considerable doctor shopping, she found one who agreed not to lecture her and simply treat the numerous lung problems she constantly develops. Her COPD prevents her from walking to work even though her Manhattan condo is only seven blocks away from the agency. Recreation such as skiing and hiking are now out of the question.

Over the next several years, her COPD progresses and she cannot even walk up a flight of stairs. She has to be hospitalized for pneumonia and shortness of breath and although she is treated well, her fierce independence makes her a difficult patient. Her doctor recommends home oxygen and that helps her. Although she is not yet 65, she qualifies for disability and therefore Medicare. Medicare pays for some home-nursing care but she has to pay for the rest. She has the good fortune to be able to afford this.

One day she becomes short of breath and is taken to the hospital where the reigning emergency room resident has her intubated minutes after setting eyes on her. Ms. Harrington is completely outraged by her state. She is dependent on a machine and finds it demeaning to use the bedpan. After several attempts, she is weaned from the respirator. Her first words question the legitimacy of the resident who intubated her.

Ms. Harrington establishes a living will and has a friend become her health care proxy. She updates her will, leaving a large portion of her estate to ecological causes. Although she is only 58, she can barely walk to the bathroom. Her doctor tells her that her FEV1 is 0.65 liter and that in his opinion, her chance of being alive two years from now is less than 20%. Ms. Harrington is rapidly losing weight as she has no appetite. Several months later, she becomes short of breath and is again is taken by ambulance to the emergency room. While there, she produces her living will informing the doctor that she does not wish to be intubated. With the use of several medications, she survives. Two months later, she has a respiratory arrest in her home and dies, joking and smoking until the end.

Comment: Ms. Harrington wisely recognized, with the help of her physician, that she was terminal. Her strong personality enabled her to assert herself so that she did not spend her final days on a respirator as so many of these poor patients do.

Case #7: Lung Cancer

Mr. Parker is a 69-year-old retired truck driver living in a modest retirement community in Florida. A true American, Mr. Parker smokes only unfiltered Camels and, while not an alcoholic, guzzles at least one beer a day. While he enjoys projecting an image of a dumb working-class stiff, he is highly intelligent and gets a sadistic delight from decimating his brother-in-law, a retired college professor, in their weekly bridge game.

Mr. Parker has little use for doctors, but a persistent cough, finally forces his hand. A chest X-ray shows a mass in his lungs and a bronchoscopy (a procedure whereby a tube is passed into the lungs) reveals that he has lung cancer. Further testing, including a CAT scan and liver-spleen scan, show no evidence of metastasis. His doctor recommends part of his lung be removed in an attempt to cure him. Mr. Parker visits the local library, becomes an expert on lung cancer, and agrees with his doctor's approach. During the surgery, his physician biopsies several lymph nodes and all are found to be negative. Thus, his doctor is cautiously optimistic.

Mr. Parker once again becomes the scourge of the bowling alley. Ten months later, while spitting, he notices blood in his saliva. A repeat chest X-ray shows the tumor has recurred.

A CAT scan and liver-spleen scan again show no evidence of metastasis. His physician recommends that the tumor be resected and that he be given radiation treatments. Mr. Parker again retreats to his local library and after considerable reading, concludes that he is going to die and there is nothing any doctor can do about it. He asks his doctor point blank if he has ever a seen a patient with recurrent lung cancer cured. His doctor says no and bluntly tells him he is going to die. He continues saying that the surgery and radiation treatment may give him several more months, but he is not even sure of that. Mr. Parker refuses all further treatment including pain medications. Four months later he passes away.

Comment: Mr. Parker made the proper decision. He may have done poorly with the second surgery in his debilitated state and no cure was possible. The average lifespan in a patient with recurrent lung cancer is about six months and treatment has never been proven to lengthen it.

Case #8: Breast Cancer

Mrs. Wethersfield is a 74-year-old widow living in suburban Los Angeles who spends her spare time gardening and visiting her grandchildren. Her gynecologist notices a breast mass on a routine physical and recommends a biopsy that proves to be breast cancer. A complete metastatic work-up is negative and a mastectomy is recommended. During the procedure, several lymph nodes in her armpit are biopsied and one of them is positive. At the recommendation of her gynecologist, she accepts one session of chemotherapy that she tolerates quite well.

Over the next several years, she develops mild hypertension but is otherwise healthy. At age 80, she starts having back pain and a bone scan and biopsy reveals that her breast cancer has metastasized. She has dramatic pain relief with hormonal therapy. Two years later, she develops hip pain. Again, a bone scan reveals metastasis but this does not respond to hormonal treatment. She attempts taking narcotics but the side effects make her too drowsy to drive. She accepts radiation therapy which diminishes the pain slightly. In the meantime, she has little appetite and starts losing weight rapidly. She is no longer able to clean her house and bathe on her own.

Mrs. Wethersfield's physician recognizes that she is entering the terminal phase of her cancer. He sees little sense in placing Mrs. Wethersfield in the hospital where she will invariably end up in intensive care hooked up to tubes and machines. Instead he recommends that she have nurses visit her house to give her injections of narcotics to control her pain and help her sleep.

Medicare pays for a large portion of this. While Mrs. Wethersfield is not wealthy, her house has appreciated and she has no intention of entering a nursing home and having the house sold to pay for it. When she dies, she wants the house sold and the proceeds split among her children. She stays in her house until she dies several months later.

Comment: Mrs. Wethersfield had a more indolent form of breast cancer and lived almost ten years after the diagnosis. This is typical of many patients and breast cancer is often a chronic disease. Her doctor was wise to recognize when she entered the terminal phase and not hospitalize her or subject her to further chemotherapy. Radiation therapy was given only for pain. Mrs. Wethersfield's refusal to go to a nursing home is entirely reasonable. She remained mentally alert and had the resources to have others help her.

Case #9: Breast Cancer

Mrs. Boswell is a 54-year-old nurse with three teenage children. Although she religiously has an annual mammogram, she notes a lump in her breast and presents to her gynecologist. A biopsy reveals that it is malignant and a liver-spleen scan shows that it already has metastasized to her liver. While she realizes that her disease is fatal, Mrs. Boswell does not want to die. She consents to aggressive chemotherapy and radiation therapy and tolerates those treatments poorly. She has multiple episodes of nausea, vomiting and loses all her hair. Her tumors diminish in size. Soon she is able to function and even insists on working.

One day, she notices some numbness in her leg. She is examined by a neurologist who orders an immediate CAT scan of her back. This reveals a large tumor impinging on her spinal cord. Aggressive radiation therapy along with steroids are given in an attempt to shrink the tumor. These modalities are unsuccessful as she becomes paralyzed and incontinent.

Mrs. Boswell is now in constant pain and narcotics offer little relief. She refuses all further treatment and is able to return to her home because her family is able to care for her. When she contracts a urinary tract infection, she refuses antibiotics and hospitalization and dies quickly.

Comment: Mrs. Boswell had a rapidly fatal form of breast cancer. No treatment was possible, but like many patients cheated out of life, she was willing to try anything. A metastasis to the spinal cord is one of the most feared complication of any cancer and palliation is often difficult. Her decision to refuse antibiotic treatment when her condition was terminal was entirely reasonable. A patient who did not have the family-support structure of Mrs. Boswell could have gone to a hospice and received outstanding and dignified care.

Case #10: Colon Cancer

Mrs. Guilford is a 66-year-old widow who develops constipation. A work-up by her physician results in the diagnosis of colon cancer and further testing shows no evidence of distant metastasis.

An attempt at a surgical cure is made. The entire tumor is removed without complications but one of her lymph nodes is positive. She accepts a session of radiation therapy and after one year is without symptoms.

However, three years later, she develops intense abdominal pain and a CAT scans reveals that the tumor has returned. Her doctor offers her further surgery but Mrs. Guilford realizes that she cannot be cured and asks only that the pain be controlled. Liberal doses of narcotics offer some relief but after several months, the pain is again intolerable. Her physician asks that she consult a pain specialist. The doctor gives her an injection that permanently deadens the nerves causing the pain and she is once again comfortable. Her condition worsens though, and she starts losing weight at a rapid rate. When she is no longer able to care for herself, she enters a hospice and passes away peacefully.

Comment: Pain control is often a problem in terminal cancer. The modality used on Mrs. Guilford is readily available and is not used enough, although it does not work in every case.

Case #: 11 AIDS

Mr. Madison is a 38-year-old gay living in suburban Atlanta. He has been HIV-positive for five years and has been taking AZT treatment for most of this time. Highly educated about his disease, he often knows more about AIDS than his doctors. His first bout with the disease comes in the form of pneumocystis pneumonia. With aggressive treatment, he survives and is discharged from the hospital and placed on maintenance antibiotics.

Mr. Madison owns a successful hair styling business and has full health insurance for his illness. When his company tried to drop him because of the high-risk nature of his profession, a letter from his attorney terminates their efforts. He has reached a rapprochement with his family, but he considers his true family to be his companion of the past three years. He makes a living will and assigns his companion to be his health care proxy.

Mr. Madison is realistic about his prognosis and has faith in his physician. He knows that his chances of being alive three years from now are slim and is determined not to become a living skeleton like so many of his friends who have died. He sells his business while he is still able to work and it is still booming. He draws up a will leaving the majority of his estate to his companion. He also establishes a modest trust fund for the education of his nephews and nieces.

When he starts to lose weight from lack of appetite, his physician offers to give him intravenous or nasogastric feedings. Mr. Madison refuses. He suffers through multiple episodes of diarrhea. Fortunately, he is not in great pain and manages to stay home. On several occasions, his physician makes a house call and assists the visiting nurse in rehydrating Mr. Madison intravenously. Mr. Madison again develops pneumocystis pneumonia. He agrees to be admitted to the hospital under the condition that he is DNR and not to be placed in intensive care. While there, he becomes confused and a CAT scan reveals multiple brain lesions. His physician explains to his companion that they could be abcesses or tumors and that he needs further testing including a spinal tap and perhaps a brain biopsy. Mr. Madison's companion refuses all diagnostic treatment. When Mr. Madison complains of a headache, he receives liberal doses of morphine. Several days later he passes away.

Comment: AIDS activists may view this scenario to be so idealized that it should be categorized as fiction. AIDS patients often die more horrible deaths with less sympathetic health care personnel and family. Nonetheless, I believe that this scenario would be more common if AIDS patients asserted themselves.

APPENDIX 1

This appendix shows the chance of those 65 and older living to be a certain age and is divided according to sex.   For example, what is the chance of a 70-year-old man living to be 90-years old?   Simply find the number 70 in the bold horizontal numbers and follow the column of numbers below it until you are across from the bold 90 in the vertical column. The answer is 17% (in bold print for demonstration). This means that of 100 men now at the age of 70, 17 of them will live to be at least 90. (Note that 1 can mean less that 1%)

MALES (Age 65 to 83)

(present age)

	65	66	67	68	69	70	71	72	73	74	75	76	77	78	79	80	81	82	83
65																			
66	98																		
67	95	97																	
68	92	95	97																
69	89	92	94	97															
70	86	89	91	94	97														
71	83	85	88	90	93	96													
72	80	82	84	86	89	92	96												
73	76	78	80	82	85	88	92	96											
74	72	74	76	78	81	84	87	91	95										
75	69	70	72	74	77	79	83	86	90	95									
76	65	66	68	70	72	75	78	81	85	89	94								
77	61	62	64	66	68	70	73	76	80	84	88	94							
78	57	58	60	61	63	65	68	71	74	78	83	88	93						
79	52	54	55	57	59	61	63	66	69	73	77	81	87	93					
80	48	50	51	52	54	56	58	61	64	67	71	75	80	85	92				
81	44	45	47	48	49	51	53	55	58	61	64	68	73	78	84	91			
82	40	41	42	43	45	46	48	50	53	55	58	62	66	71	76	83	91		
83	36	37	38	39	40	42	43	45	47	50	52	56	59	63	68	74	81	90	
84	32	33	34	35	36	37	38	40	42	44	46	49	53	56	61	66	72	80	89
85	28	29	29	30	31	32	34	35	37	39	41	43	46	49	53	58	63	70	78
86	25	26	27	27	28	29	30	32	33	35	37	39	42	45	48	52	57	63	70
87	22	23	24	24	25	26	27	28	30	31	33	35	37	40	43	47	51	56	63
88	20	20	21	22	22	23	24	25	26	27	29	31	33	35	38	41	45	50	55
89	17	18	18	19	19	20	21	22	23	24	25	27	29	31	33	36	39	43	48
90	15	15	16	16	17	17	18	19	20	21	22	23	25	27	29	31	34	38	42
91	13	13	14	14	14	15	15	16	17	18	19	20	21	23	24	27	29	32	36
92	11	11	11	12	12	13	13	14	14	15	16	17	18	19	21	22	25	27	30
93	9	9	10	10	10	10	11	11	12	12	13	14	15	16	17	19	20	23	25
94	7	8	8	8	8	9	9	9	10	10	11	11	12	13	14	15	17	19	21
95	6	6	6	7	7	7	7	8	8	8	9	9	10	11	11	12	14	15	17
96	5	5	5	5	5	6	6	6	6	7	7	7	8	8	9	10	11	12	13
97	4	4	4	4	4	4	5	5	5	5	6	6	7	7	8	8	9	10	
98	3	3	3	3	3	3	4	4	4	4	4	5	5	5	6	6	7	8	
99	2	2	2	2	2	3	3	3	3	3	3	4	4	4	4	5	5	6	
100	2	2	2	2	2	2	2	2	2	2	3	3	3	3	4	4	4		
101	1	1	1	1	1	1	1	1	1	2	2	2	2	2	2	3	3		
102	1	1	1	1	1	1	1	1	1	1	1	1	1	2	2	2	2		
103	1	1	1	1	1	1	1	1	1	1	1	1	1	1	1	1	1		
104	1	1	1	1	1	1	1	1	1	1	1	1	1	1	1	1	1		
105	1	1	1	1	1	1	1	1	1	1	1	1	1	1	1	1	1		

MALES (Age 84 to 104)

	84	85	86	87	88	89	90	91	92	93	94	95	96	97	98	99	100	101	102	103	104
85	88																				
86	79	87																			
87	71	78	87																		
88	62	69	78	87																	
89	55	61	69	77	86																
90	47	53	60	67	76	86															
91	40	45	51	57	65	74	85														
92	34	38	43	48	55	62	72	84													
93	28	32	36	50	46	52	60	70	83												
94	23	26	30	33	37	43	49	58	68	82											
95	19	21	24	27	30	35	40	47	55	66	81										
96	15	17	19	21	24	28	32	37	44	53	64	80									
97	12	13	15	17	19	21	25	29	34	41	50	62	78								
98	9	10	11	13	14	16	19	22	26	32	38	48	60	77							
99	7	7	8	10	11	12	14	17	20	24	29	36	45	57	75						
100	5	5	6	7	8	9	10	12	14	17	21	26	33	42	55	73					
101	4	4	4	5	6	6	7	9	10	12	15	18	23	30	39	52	71				
102	3	3	3	3	4	4	5	6	7	8	10	13	16	20	26	35	48	68			
103	2	2	2	2	2	3	3	4	5	5	7	8	10	13	17	23	32	45	66		
104	1	1	1	1	2	2	2	3	3	4	3	7	8	11	15	20	28	41	63		
105	1	1	1	1	1	1	1	2	2	2	2	4	5	6	9	12	17	25	37	59	

FEMALES (Age 65 to 84)

	65	66	67	68	69	70	71	72	73	74	75	76	77	78	79	80	81	82	83	84
66	99																			
67	97	98																		
68	96	97	98																	
69	94	95	97	98																
70	92	93	95	96	98															
71	90	91	93	94	96	98														
72	88	89	91	92	94	96	98													
73	86	87	88	90	91	93	95	97												
74	83	85	86	87	89	91	93	96	97											
75	81	82	83	85	86	88	90	92	94	97										
76	78	79	81	82	83	85	87	89	91	94	97									
77	75	76	78	79	80	82	84	86	88	90	93	96								
78	72	73	74	76	77	79	80	82	84	87	90	93	96							
79	69	70	71	73	74	75	77	79	81	83	86	89	92	96						
80	66	67	68	69	70	72	73	75	77	79	82	84	88	91	95					
81	62	63	64	65	67	68	69	71	73	75	77	80	83	86	90	95				
82	58	60	61	62	63	64	65	67	69	71	73	75	78	81	85	89	94			
83	55	56	57	57	59	60	61	62	64	66	68	70	73	76	79	83	88	93		
84	51	52	52	53	54	55	56	58	59	61	63	65	67	70	73	77	81	86	93	
85	47	47	48	49	50	51	52	53	54	56	58	60	62	64	67	71	75	79	85	92
86	43	43	44	45	46	47	48	49	50	52	53	55	57	60	62	65	69	73	79	85
87	40	40	41	41	42	43	44	45	46	48	49	50	53	55	57	60	63	67	72	78
88	36	37	37	38	38	39	40	41	42	43	45	46	48	50	52	55	58	61	66	71
89	32	33	33	34	34	35	36	37	38	39	40	41	43	45	47	49	52	55	59	64
90	29	29	29	30	30	31	32	33	33	34	35	36	38	40	41	43	46	49	52	56
91	25	25	26	26	27	27	28	28	29	30	31	32	33	35	36	38	40	43	46	49
92	22	22	22	23	23	23	24	25	25	26	27	28	29	30	31	33	35	37	39	42
93	19	19	19	19	20	20	20	21	21	22	23	24	24	25	27	28	29	31	33	36
94	15	16	16	16	16	17	17	18	18	18	19	20	20	21	22	23	25	26	28	30
95	13	13	13	13	14	14	14	14	15	15	15	16	17	18	18	19	20	22	23	25
96	10	10	11	11	11	11	11	12	12	12	13	13	14	14	15	16	17	18	19	20
97	8	8	9	9	9	9	9	9	10	10	10	11	11	11	12	13	13	14	15	16
98	6	6	7	7	7	7	7	8	8	8	9	9	9	10	10	11	12	13		
99	5	5	5	5	5	5	6	6	6	6	6	6	7	7	7	8	8	9	9	10
100	4	4	4	4	4	4	4	5	5	5	5	6	6	6	6	7	7	8		
101	3	3	3	3	3	3	3	3	3	4	4	4	4	4	4	5	5	5	5	5
102	2	2	2	2	2	2	2	2	2	2	3	3	3	3	3	3	4	4	4	
103	1	1	1	2	2	2	2	2	2	2	2	2	2	2	2	2	2	3	3	
104	1	1	1	1	1	1	1	1	1	1	1	1	1	1	1	1	2	2	2	
105	1	1	1	1	1	1	1	1	1	1	1	1	1	1	1	1	1	1	1	1

FEMALES (Age 85-104)

	85	86	87	88	89	90	91	92	93	94	95	96	97	98	99	100	101	102	103	104
86	92																			
87	85	92																		
88	77	83	91																	
89	69	75	81	90																
90	61	66	72	80	89															
91	54	55	63	70	78	87														
92	46	50	55	60	67	75	86													
93	39	43	46	51	57	64	73	85												
94	33	36	39	43	48	54	62	71	84											
95	27	29	32	35	39	44	51	59	69	83										
96	22	23	26	29	32	36	41	48	56	67	81									
97	17	19	21	23	26	29	33	38	45	54	65	80								
98	14	15	17	18	20	23	26	30	36	42	51	63	79							
99	11	12	13	14	16	18	20	23	28	33	40	49	61	78						
100	8	9	10	11	12	13	15	18	21	25	30	37	47	59	76					
101	6	7	7	8	9	10	11	13	16	17	23	28	35	44	57	74				
102	4	5	5	6	6	7	8	10	11	14	16	20	25	32	41	54	72			
103	3	3	4	4	5	5	6	7	8	9	11	14	18	22	29	38	51	70		
104	2	2	2	3	3	3	4	5	5	6	8	10	12	15	20	27	34	48	67	
105	1	1	2	2	2	2	3	3	3	4	5	6	8	10	13	16	22	31	44	60

APPENDIX 2

SIMPLIFIED SUMMARY OF EACH STATES LAWS REGARDING TERMINAL CARE

Listed below is the status of terminal-care legislation in each state as of 1991. Some statements are vague because there is no consensus. Legal scholars themselves may disagree on the ramifications and interpretations of the laws and judicial opinions of the various states. Updated information is available from:

> The Society for the Right to Die
> 250 West 57th Street
> New York, NY 10107
> 212-246-6962

ALABAMA
- recognizes a living will
- no specific legislation recognizing a health care proxy
- may remove a respirator and tube feedings in certain medical conditions

ALASKA
- recognizes a living will
- permits a health care proxy (via durable power of attorney) to consent to treatment but there is no specific statute regarding the withdrawal of a respirator or tube feeding
- can withdraw or withhold both respirator and tube feeding under certain medical conditions

ARIZONA
- recognizes a living will
- health care proxy can (via durable power of attorney) withdraw tube feedings and respirator
- can withdraw or withhold tube feeding but judicial interpretation is necessary

ARKANSAS
- recognizes a living will
- living will recognizes a health care proxy that can withdraw a respirator and tube feedings
- can withdraw or withhold tube feeding under certain medical conditions

CALIFORNIA
- recognizes a living will
- health care proxy (via durable power of attorney) can withdraw tube feedings and a respirator
- may remove a respirator and tube feeding in under certain medical conditions

COLORADO
- recognizes a living will
- health care proxy (via durable power of attorney) can withdraw tube feedings and a respirator
- may withhold or withdraw tube feedings under certain medical conditions

CONNECTICUT
- recognizes a living will
- health care proxy can withdraw a respirator and tube feedings
- may withhold or withdraw tube feeding and respirator under certain medical conditions

DELAWARE
- recognizes a living will
- health care proxy can make medical decisions
- may remove a respirator but there is no specific mention of tube feedings

FLORIDA
- recognizes a living will (and those from other states)
- health care proxy can withdraw a respirator and tube feedings
- may withhold or withdraw tube feedings under certain medical conditions

GEORGIA
- recognizes a living will
- health care proxy (via durable power of attorney) can remove a respirator
- may withhold or withdraw tube feeding according to the judiciary but not according to the legislature

HAWAII
- recognizes a living will
- health care proxy (via durable power of attorney) can withdraw a respirator or tube feedings
- withdrawal of a respirator and tube feedings is subject to judicial interpretation

IDAHO
- recognizes a living will
- health care proxy can withdraw a respirator and tube feedings
- may withdraw tube feedings and respirator under certain medical conditions

ILLINOIS
- recognizes a living will
- health care proxy (via durable power of attorney) can withdraw a respirator or tube feedings
- may withdraw tube feedings and a respirator

INDIANA
- recognizes a living will
- health care proxy may make medical decisions but removal of a respirator or tube feedings may require judicial approval
- need judicial approval to withdraw a respirator or tube feeding

IOWA
- recognizes a living will
- health care proxy (via durable power of attorney) may decide to withdraw respirator or tube feedings in certain situations
- judicial or legislative interpretation sometimes needed before withdrawing a feeding tube or respirator

KANSAS
- recognizes a living
- health care proxy may decide to withdraw respirator or tube feedings in certain situations
- may withdraw tube feedings and a respirator

KENTUCKY
- recognizes a living will
- health care proxy (via durable power of attorney) can withdraw a respirator but not necessarily tube feedings
- tube feeding required in some circumstances

LOUISIANA
- recognizes a living will
- health care proxy (via durable power of attorney) can make medical decisions but there is no specific authorization regarding tube feedings
- can remove a respirator but there is no specific mention of tube feedings

MAINE
- recognizes a living will
- health care proxy can withdraw a respirator or tube feedings
- may withdraw tube feedings or a respirator

MARYLAND
- recognizes a living will
- health care proxy (via durable power of attorney) can withdraw respirator and tube feedings
- judicial interpretation necessary to withhold or withdraw tube feedings

MASSACHUSETTS
- recognizes a living will
- health care proxy (via durable power of attorney) can withdraw respirator and tube feedings
- may withdraw tube feedings or a respirator

MICHIGAN
- recognizes a living will
- health care proxy (via durable power of attorney) can withdraw respirator and tube feedings
- may withdraw tube feedings or a respirator

MINNESOTA
- recognizes a living will
- living will recognizes a health care proxy that can withdraw a respirator and tube feedings
- may withdraw tube feedings or a respirator

MISSOURI
- recognizes a living will
- no specific legislation recognizing a health care proxy
- tube feedings required in some cases and withholding and withdrawing tube feedings and a respirator is prohibited in some circumstances [state of Nancy Cruzan]

MONTANA
- recognizes a living will
- no specific legislation recognizing a health care proxy
- may withdraw tube feedings or a respirator

NEBRASKA
- does not recognize a living will or health care proxy

NEVADA
- recognizes a living will
- health care proxy (via durable power of attorney) can withdraw tube feedings or respirator
- may withdraw tube feedings or a respirator

NEW HAMPSHIRE
- recognizes a living will
- no specific legislation recognizing a health care proxy
- judicial interpretation may be necessary to withdraw tube feedings or a respirator

NEW JERSEY
- recognizes a living will
- health care proxy via durable power of attorney may withdraw tube feedings or a respirator
- may withdraw tube feedings or respirator

NEW MEXICO
- recognizes a living will
- health care proxy (via durable power or attorney) may consent to treatment but has not specific power to remove a feeding tube or respirator
- may withdraw respirator but present laws have no specific mention of tube feedings

NEW YORK
- recognizes a living will
- health care proxy (via durable power or attorney) may withdraw respirator or tube feeding
- may withdraw tube feedings or respirator

NORTH CAROLINA
- recognizes a living will
- health care proxy (via durable power or attorney) may consent to treatment but has not specific power to remove a feeding tube or respirator
- may withdraw tube feedings or respirator

NORTH DAKOTA
- recognizes a living will
- no specific legislation regarding a health care proxy
- may withdraw tube feedings or respirator

OHIO
- recognizes a living will
- health care proxy (via durable power of attorney) can withdraw tube feedings or respirator
- may withdraw tube feedings or a respirator but not in all circumstances

OKLAHOMA
- recognizes a living will
- no specific legislation regarding a health care proxy
- may withdraw tube feedings or respirator but they may be required in some circumstances

OREGON
- recognizes a living will
- health care proxy (via durable power of attorney) can withdraw tube feedings or respirator
- may withdraw tube feedings or a respirator

PENNSYLVANIA
- living will legislation pending
- health care proxy (via durable power of attorney) may consent to treatment but no specific power to withdraw tube feedings or respirator
- may withdraw tube feedings or respirator

RHODE ISLAND
- recognizes a living will
- health care proxy (via durable power of attorney) can withdraw tube feedings or respirator
- may withdraw tube feedings or respirator

SOUTH DAKOTA
- recognizes a living will
- health care proxy (via durable power of attorney) can withdraw tube feedings or respirator
- may withdraw tube feedings or respirator

TENNESSEE
- recognizes a living will
- health care proxy (via durable power of attorney) can withdraw tube feedings or respirator
- may withdraw tube feedings or respirator

TEXAS
- recognizes a living will
- health care proxy (via durable power of attorney) can withdraw tube feedings or respirator
- may withdraw life support a respirator but no specific mention of tube feedings

UTAH
- recognizes a living will
- health care proxy recognized by no specific power to withdraw a respirator or tube feedings
- judicial or legislative interpretation necessary to withdraw tube feedings or respirator

VERMONT
- recognizes a living will
- health care proxy (via durable power of attorney) can withdraw tube feedings or respirator
- may remove a respirator but present laws do not specifically mention of tube feedings

VIRGINIA
- recognizes a living will
- health care proxy (via durable power of attorney) can withdraw tube feedings or respirator
- may remove life support or respirator but judicial interpretation sometimes required to withdraw or withhold tube feedings

WASHINGTON
- living will recognized
- health care proxy (via durable power of attorney) may consent to treatment but no specific power to withdraw tube feedings or respirator
- may remove a respirator but withdrawing tube feeding restricted

WEST VIRGINIA
- living will recognized
- health care proxy (via durable power of attorney) may withdraw tube feedings or respirator
- judicial or legislative interpretation may be required to withdraw tube feeding or respirator

WISCONSIN
- living will recognized
- health care proxy (via durable power of attorney) may withdraw tube feedings or respirator
- may withdraw respirator or tube feedings

Index

Coumadin, 78
CPR, 16, 19, 51
Cruzan, Nancy, 3, 54
Cryptococcal Meningitis, 146

Dementia, 58 - 59, 61
Depression, 64, 80
Dialysis, 21, 91
DNR, 19, 151
DRG's, 37
Drug Overdose, 75
Dukes' Staging of Colon Cancer, 114
Durable Power of Attorney, 44

Ejection Fraction, 89, 93
Electrocardiogram, 88
Emphysema - See also COPD
Endometrial Cancer, 132
Esophageal Cancer, 127
Estate Taxes, 42 - 43
Euthanasia, 41

Feeding Tube - See also Artificial Nutrition
FEV1, 97 - 98, 101, 160

Glioma, 125 - See also Brain Cancer
Guardianship, 44

Harvard Definition of Brain Death - See also Brain Death
Hayflick Principle, 10
Head Trauma, 75
Health Care Proxy, 48, 51, 53 - 56, 66, 80, 150
Heart Attack, 87, 89
Heart Disease - See Coronary Artery Disease
Heparin, 78
Hodgkin's Disease, 103, 107
Home Care, 29, 40
Hospice, 29, 40 - 41, 101, 152

Hyperalimentation - See also Artificial nutrition
Hypothermia, 75

Incontinence, 24, 67
Inheritance Taxes - See also Estate Taxes
Intubation, 92, 101

Joint Ownership, 46

Kidney Cancer, 128

Leukemia, 103
Life Insurance, 42
Life Span, 9, 12, 25
Liver Cancer, 127
Living Trust, 46
Living Will, 48 - 50, 54, 66
Long-Term Care Insurance, 39 - 40
Long-Term Health Care, 32, 36, 39
Lumpectomy, 117
Lung Cancer, 106, 111 - 112, 124, 160 - 161
Lymphomas, 146

Mastectomy, 117
Meals-On-Wheels, 33
Medicaid, 27, 31, 35 - 37, 148, 154
Medicare, 27 - 28, 30 - 33, 37, 41, 47, 149
Medigap, 31
Memory, 61 - 62
Metastatic Cancer, 62
Multi-Infarct Dementia, 68 - 69

Nasogastric tube - See also Artificial nutrition
National Practioner's Data Bank, 49
Nitroglycerin, 85
Nursing Home, 32, 34

Ovarian Cancer, 130 - 131

Pain Control, 109
Pancreatic Cancer, 127
Parkinson's Disease, 69 - 70
Persistent Vegetative State, 50 - 51
Pneumocystis Pneumonia, 144
Power of Attorney, 44
Prostate Cancer, 119 - 121, 123

Quinlan, Karen Ann, 3, 20,74

Radiation Therapy, 107
Rehabilitation, 78
Renal Cell Cancer - See Kidney Cancer
Representative Payee, 46
Respirator, 19, 51, 54, 74, 92
Retirement Community, 33

Self-Awareness, 22, 80
Spirometer, 96
Staging, 107
Stomach Cancer, 127
Stress Test, 83
Strokes, 57, 71, 77, 79, 81, 155 - 158

Terminal Cancer Syndrome, 108 - 109
Terminal Disease, 21, 25
Testicular cancer, 103
TIA, 77
Trusts, 43

Uterine Cancer - See Endometrial Cancer

Ventilation- See also Respirator

Will To Live, 22 - 25
Wills, 43, 150

ORDER FORM

Michelle Publishing Company
2317 Silas Deane Highway
Rocky Hill, CT 06067
203-721-8800 (Office)   203-721-1694 (Fax)

Number of Copies	Price per Copy
1	$13.95
2-5	$11.95
5-9	$10.95
10-99	$9.95
100 and over	$8.95

Please send me_____ copies of *When To Refuse Treatment*. Please include $1.50 postage and handling for one book and 50¢ per book for two or more not to exceed $7.50. Prices subject to change without notice. Add 20% for Canada. Do not send cash.

NAME_____

ADDRESS_____

CITY_____ STATE/ZIP_____

__CK ENCL   __VISA   __MC

Card#_____ Exp Date:_____

Signature _____